Creating a
Caring Science Curriculum
An Emancipatory Pedagogy
for Nursing

Marcia Hills, PhD, RN, is the Director and President of the Canadian Consortium for Health Promotion Research, and Professor of Nursing at University of Victoria, Canada. She has been actively engaged in research and evaluation for over 20 years, is the Principal Investigator on two federally funded (Canadian Institutes for Health Research) multiyear research initiatives, and is the Co-Investigator on five additional projects. She presents at numerous conferences in Canada, the United States, and abroad.

Dr. Hills is an elected member of the Board of Trustees for the International Union for Health Promotion and Education (IUHPE) and a member of the North American Regional Office (NARO). As part of her work with these organizations, she was a member of the Steering Committee for the IUHPE Global Program on Effectiveness, co-chaired the NARO Effectiveness Working Group, and was VP for the Organization of the World Conference, and Cochair of the 2007 World Conference on Health Promotion and Health Education, as held in Vancouver in 2007. Recently, Dr. Hills was invited to join a World Health Organization working group led by Erio Ziglio to develop an international project on evaluating health assets in partnership with Health Canada, the Health Development Agency (UK), and the Centers for Disease Control (Atlanta, Georgia, USA).

Jean Watson, PhD, RN, AHN-BC, FAAN, is Distinguished Professor of Nursing and former Dean of the School of Nursing at the University of Colorado. She is founder of the Center for Human Caring in Colorado, a Fellow of the American Academy of Nursing, and past-president of the National League for Nursing.

Dr. Watson has earned undergraduate and graduate degrees in nursing and psychiatric-mental health nursing with a PhD in educational psychology and counseling. She is a widely published author and recipient of several awards and honors, including an international Kellogg Fellowship in Australia, a Fulbright Research Award in Sweden, and nine honorary doctoral degrees, such as Honorary International Doctor of Science awards from Goteborg University in Sweden and from Luton University in London.

Clinical nurses and academic programs throughout the world use her published works on the philosophy and theory of human caring and the art and science of caring in nursing. Dr. Watson's caring philosophy is used to guide new models of caring and healing practices in diverse settings worldwide.

At the University of Colorado, Dr. Watson holds the title of Distinguished Professor of Nursing, the highest honor accorded to its faculty for scholarly work. In 1998–1999 she assumed that nation's first endowed chair in Caring Science, based at the University of Colorado.

Creating a
Caring Science Curriculum

An Emancipatory Pedagogy
for Nursing

Marcia Hills, PhD, RN

Jean Watson, PhD, RN, AHN-BC, FAAN

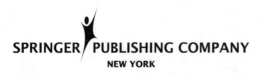

SPRINGER PUBLISHING COMPANY
NEW YORK

Watson Caring
Science Institute

Springer Publishing Company, LLC
11 West 42nd Street
New York, NY 10036
www.springerpub.com

Acquisitions Editor: Allan Graubard
Senior Editor: Rose Mary Piscitelli
Composition: Nandini Loganathan/S4Carlisle Publishing Services

ISBN: 978-0-8261-0589-9
E-book ISBN: 978-0-8261-0590-5

11 12 13 14/ 5 4 3 2 1

The author and the publisher of this Work have made every effort to use sources believed to be reliable to provide information that is accurate and compatible with the standards generally accepted at the time of publication. Because medical science is continually advancing, our knowledge base continues to expand. Therefore, as new information becomes available, changes in procedures become necessary. We recommend that the reader always consult current research and specific institutional policies before performing any clinical procedure. The author and publisher shall not be liable for any special, consequential, or exemplary damages resulting, in whole or in part, from the readers' use of, or reliance on, the information contained in this book. The publisher has no responsibility for the persistence or accuracy of URLs for external or third-party Internet Web sites referred to in this publication and does not guarantee that any content on such Web sites is, or will remain, accurate or appropriate.

Library of Congress Cataloging-in-Publication Data
Hills, Marcia.
  Creating a caring curriculum: an emancipatory pedagogy for nursing / Marcia Hills, Jean Watson.
    p. cm.
  ISBN 978-0-8261-0589-9
 1. Nursing — Study and teaching.   2. Curriculum planning.   I. Watson, Jean, 1940-
 II. Title.
  RT71.H545 2011
  610.73076 — dc22   2011008090

Printed in the United States of America by Bang Printing

*T*his book is dedicated to Em Olivia Bevis—mentor, colleague, master teacher, leader, visionary and loving person, and personal friend to us and thousands of others. A loving and provocative teacher, she dared you to reach the threshold of your own mind by challenging your taken-for-granted assumptions in a way that opened your heart and soul to new learning. Em often captured the imagination of hundreds of nurse educators crowded into a room to hear her speak. Her brilliance was in leading them back to themselves through critical questioning and dialogue with their colleagues, not necessarily with her.

She died too young and is deeply missed by her colleagues and friends and the nursing profession that didn't have enough time to sit in her presence. Writing this book is a way to continue her legacy and a way to keep her vision for nursing and nursing education alive and vibrant.

Em loved nursing, and she loved nursing education more. Her words below echo her deep commitment to this wonderful profession. She writes:

> There is a compelling splendor about both teaching and nursing that demands the highest form of endeavor, for their ends are linked to the magnificent miracle of human thought and human life.
>
> They have a common core of caring about the human condition and an obligation to its improvement that confers a radiant beauty on the meanest of tasks in their service.
>
> They are a societal trust.
>
> And for those that combine these two tasks into the teaching of nursing, there is a moral commitment to society's needs that requires industrious constancy in self-development efforts so that this trust will be steadfastly and excellently honored.
>
> *(Bevis, 1989, p. 153)*

CONTENTS

CONTRIBUTORS

ANNE BOYKIN, PhD, RN   Professor and Dean, Christine E. Lynn College of Nursing, Florida Atlantic University, Boca Raton, Florida

MARY ENZMAN HINES, RN, PhD, CNS, CPNP, AHN-BC   President, American Holistic Nurses Association (AHNA), Certified Pediatric Nurse Practitioner, Colorado Springs Health Partners, Colorado Springs, Colorado

MARY ROCKWOOD LANE, PhD, RN, FAAN   Associate Faculty, WCSI, Associate Professor, College of Nursing, Faculty Associate, Watson Caring Science Institute, University of Florida, Gainesville, Florida

SHEILA LEWIS, MHSc, BScN, CHTP   School of Nursing, Faculty of Health, York University, Toronto, Canada

RAHEL NAEF, MN, RN   Cantonal Hospital Lucerne, Toronto, Canada

MARTHA ROGERS, EdD, MScN, RN   Alkinson Faculty of Liberal and Professional Studies and School of Nursing, Faculty of Health, York University, Toronto, Canada

MICHAEL SAMUELS, MD   Director, Art as a Healing Force, Bolinas, California

KATHLEEN L. SITZMAN, MS, RN, PhD   Associate Professor of Nursing, Weber State University, Ogden, Utah

MARLAINE C. SMITH, RN, PhD, AHN-BC, FAAN   Helen K. Persson Eminent Scholar and Associate Dean for Academic Programs, Christine E. Lynn College of Nursing, Florida Atlantic University, Boca Raton, Florida

THERIS A. TOUHY, DNP, CNS   Professor, Christine E. Lynn College of Nursing, Florida Atlantic University, Boca Raton, Florida

FOREWORD

D
R. MARCIA HILLS AND DR. JEAN WATSON have written an innovative and thoughtful curriculum guide for making visible and creating a curriculum around Caring Science. They recognize that such a curriculum will require emancipatory pedagogies in order to critically reflect on what impedes the development of a curriculum that focuses on the core disciplinary knowledge, skills, and practices of caring. They wisely adopt an inclusive view of science, enlarging the scope of scientific inquiry into the human sciences, and in particular the human science of caring.

The book is permeated with a conversational and dialogical tone to encourage reflective thought about its stance and aims. The actual examples drawn from colleges and departments of nursing that have developed a Caring Science–based curriculum are helpful in laying out the assumptions, structures, and goals of a Caring Science Curriculum. They purposefully blur the distinctions between art and science with the goal of enlarging the view of science to take up and learn from art in addition to experimental research. The authors discuss the confusion over boundaries and qualitative distinctions between medicine and nursing. They are not timid about addressing "sacred cows" like evidence-based practice. Not everyone will agree with their premises and assertions, but all will confront the need to think deeply and anew on how to bring caring practices in from the margins of nursing as a science and practice.

The authors state in the first chapter:

> A Caring Science curriculum seeks to create authentic, egalitarian, human-to-human relationships. This assumption is based on the notion that there is reciprocity between power, knowledge, and control, and that, in order for there to be more equitable relationships, those with power need to give up/share control, so that others may benefit and share their knowledge, thus their power.

> Authentic power is shared power; it is power with, not power over. (p. 17, Chapter 1)

This book has high aims and sometimes gets caught up in oppositional comparisons that clash with the collaborative and relational harmony goals of the work in their critique of traditional Allopathic medicine and Rational Empirical Science. Nevertheless, this is a significant work, calling nurses to move their caring science and work in from the margins. The value and centrality of human caring are affirmed. It is impossible to read this work without thinking new thoughts and envisioning new possibilities for nursing as a discipline.

Patricia Benner, RN, PhD, FAAN

PREFACE

W E WROTE THIS BOOK IN RESPONSE to a perception that the curriculum revolution, a hallmark event in nursing education in the late 1980s and early 1990s, had yet to fulfill its mandate to reform nursing education to embrace a human caring science perspective. Some progress has been made, but there is still much to accomplish. This book is intended to provoke further debate and discussion about Caring Science as the foundation and philosophy of nursing and to explore emancipatory approaches to pedagogy as a way to move the nursing education agenda forward in its search for clarity of its foundation as a mature discipline.

This book is not a "theory" book nor is it a "how to" book. We have attempted to present material in way that inspires further and deeper thinking about a topic. The purpose is to engage critical thinking and reflection and to assist both teachers and students to develop their own way of teaching and learning within the context of a Caring Science curriculum.

The book is structured in five Units consisting of several chapters each. The Unit overview introduces the chapters that are within it and the concepts covered in each chapter. Each chapter is structured to maximize student engagement by providing reflective exercises, called "Time Out for Reflection," and structured learning activities that encourage the integration of theory and practice into the learning process. Also, students are requested to create learning groups or partners so that they can engage in critical dialogue while learning from the text. Finally, students are encouraged to keep a learning journal that is intended to stimulate personal reflection within the learning process. Taken together, these processes are intended to kindle a deeper level of reflection and engagement that inspires and inspirits the intersection between the personal and the professional in teaching and learning.

Marcia Hills, PhD, RN
Jean Watson, PhD, RN, AHN-BC, FAAN

ACKNOWLEDGMENTS

From Marcia

THE FIRST PERSON THAT I WANT to acknowledge is Em Olivia Bevis. She was my mentor, friend, and godmother to my son, Benny. She taught me to have courage in the face of adversity, and she inspired me to dedicate my career to nursing education. My husband, John, has been a "rock" for me. Not only has he been encouraging and supportive, but he has read and edited the entire manuscript several times. I am sure that we caused him many headaches, but he rarely complained and gave lovingly of his time and his talents. My children, Jenna and Benny, were supportive and encouraging and really understood when I had to miss time with them to work on this book. To my students and colleagues from whom I have learned so much, I thank you for your patience and for providing me space when I needed to work on this manuscript. And, to my friend and colleague, Jean Watson, thank you for the opportunity and the love we have shared in this joint endeavor, always keeping Em's and your vision from your original book, *Toward a Caring Curriculum*, close to our hearts so that we could contribute to the dream that Nursing will claim its rightful place as a Caring Science. Thanks for the journey!

Finally, I want to acknowledge Springer Publishing Company, especially Allan Graubard, Executive Editor, and Elizabeth Stump, Assistant Editor. Your support and encouragement never faltered even when my confidence wavered. Thank you.

From Jean

THIS WORK ACKNOWLEDGES AND HONORS EM, and the magical happenings of the earlier era of the writings, workshops, seminars, conferences, and curriculum activities sparked by NLN. I celebrate the joy of participating in the cocreated activities with Em and Marcia, Chris Tanner, Joyce Murray, and hundreds of others during the era of the caring curriculum revolution.

I acknowledge and pay tribute to the passing of time that has sustained aspects of the sparks of that "revolution" but now is opening to a longing and a possible flame of interest for a new evolutionary era. I am deeply appreciative of the learning and teachings of and with Em; of the conferences and workshops in Canada and the United States with Em, Marcia, and others. I am grateful for Marcia and her leadership in this book, bringing forth another turn from the origins that spawned this evolution for a caring science curriculum. I think Em, looking down upon us, is excited and celebrating, radiating her big loving smile on nursing and this continuing work. The book and its energy are influenced, inspired, and dedicated to Em, and our hope for her lasting legacy. My continuing gratitude goes to Allan Graubard for his support and guidance on the original book, and his enduring support for this next phase of nursing education.

I
FOUNDATIONS OF A CARING SCIENCE CURRICULUM

I N THIS UNIT, WE LAY the foundations for a Caring Science Curriculum. We argue that a Caring Science curriculum offers a new disciplinary discourse. This work offers the next evolution in professional nursing education; it places humanity, human evolution, human caring, health, and healing as its foundation. A Caring Science curriculum honors and celebrates diversity among the students-teachers and among approaches to teaching and learning. It is a revolution for whole person teaching, learning, and knowing. It invites joy, a liberated human spirit, and passionate interest back into our lives and learning. It moves us toward a transformative consciousness of whole person learning as the preferred pedagogical orientation and practices. Unit 1 has two chapters.

In Chapter 1, Caring Science: Curriculum Revolutions and Detours Along the Way, we articulate the difference between the **discipline** of nursing and the **profession** of nursing and describe why understanding these differences is critical in developing a Caring Science curriculum. In addition, we describe the underlying philosophy and theory of Caring Science and its implications for developing a Caring Science curriculum.

In Chapter 2, Beliefs and Assumptions: The Hidden Drivers of Curriculum Development, we describe the underlying beliefs and assumptions that are intrinsic to a Caring Science Curriculum. In addition, we introduce some key concepts that are explored further in future chapters.

1
Caring Science: Curriculum Revolutions and Detours Along the Way

What about a model that inspires? That shows us what we would like to become, and infuses us with the ideas and strength needed to approximate it.
—*Smith, 1982*

I T HAS BEEN MORE THAN 20 years now since the National League of Nursing (NLN) began to call for reform in nursing educa- tion, a movement that has come to be known as the Curriculum Revolution. This was a significant time in the history of nursing educa- tion in the United States as nursing leaders banded together to deinsti- tutionalize the long-standing behaviorist, Tylerian model of education that nursing education had been entrenched in for more than 40 years.

This revolution called for a paradigm shift in nursing educa- tion from behaviorism and empiricism to human science and caring as foundations upon which to create nursing curricula (Bevis, 1988; Moccia, 1988; Munhall, 1988; Tanner, 1988; Watson, 1988). It demanded new pedagogies that created transformational learning and curricu- lum design that focused on critical thinking, problem-solving, and learning, rather than on content to be transmitted. It challenged nursing educators to aspire to graduate nurses who were not only technically competent, but whose practice was steeped in the values and ethics of caring as the moral obligation of nursing to society.

Yet in 2003, the NLN confirmed that much of the innovation sought had focused instead on the addition or rearrangement of traditional content within the curriculum where we "switch, swap and slide content around" (Bevis, 1988, p. 27; Tanner, 2003).

In 2008, *Advances in Nursing Science* published a volume on the topic of the discipline of nursing. In this issue, it was noted by Newman, Smith, Pharris, and Jones (2008) that the discipline is in a transfor- mative phase. Moreover, it was reasserted here that within "the *disci- pline* of nursing, the concepts of health, caring, consciousness, mutual

3

process, patterning, presence, and meaning, . . . are essential to nursing" (Newman et al., 2008; in Smith & McCarthy, 2010, p. 46). Further, Smith and McCarthy's (2010) recent comprehensive review of seminal documents "guiding the development of baccalaureate and higher degree educational curriculum in nursing" (American Association of Colleges of Nursing [AACN], 2006, 2007, 2008) concluded: "nursing knowledge consisting of the philosophies, theories, research and practice models of the *discipline was mentioned tangentially, not centrally, and rarely explicitly*" ([our italics] p. 49). Others (Cowling, Smith, & Watson, 2008; Willis, Grace, & Roy, 2008) have defined similar meanings attesting to the disciplinary foundation of nursing, which include the human dimensions, consciousness, caring, relationships, and so on. **So, what happened to the curriculum revolution?**

DETOURS ALONG THE WAY

We will examine three areas to explain the detours that drew us away from the caring curriculum revolution and inhibit nursing evolving within its disciplinary foundation:

- The false dichotomy of nursing as an art and a science
- The ambivalent and tormented relationship between nursing science and medical science
- Nursing's fascination with evidence-based practice (EBP).

Nursing as an Art and a Science: A False Dichotomy

> Nursing is an art, and if it is to be made an art, it requires as exclusive a devotion and as hard a preparation as any painter's or sculptor's work; for what is having to do with a dead canvas or cold marble, compared to having to do with the living body—the temple of God's spirit? It is one of the fine arts: I would say the finest of the Fine Arts.
>
> (Nightingale, 1860)

As famous as Nightingale's quote of "nursing as an art . . . the finest of the Fine Arts" is, it has had a conflicting and paradoxical impact on nursing as a mature distinct discipline. Nursing's scientific evolution has tended to create an either/or approach to art and science—resulting in a false dichotomy between art and science: thus separating caring out as "art" and medical–empirical-procedural aspects as "science." This false dichotomy stands in contrast to a human Caring Science model within a disciplinary framework, which seeks to embrace and integrate both. As Smith (1993) states: "Science is considered as quantifiable, covering the nurse's science of curing and treating illness whereas arts are considered expressive, covering nurse's art of healing" (p. 42). This notion is explained further by Castledine (2010) when he states: "The scientific components of medicine have also become the scientific aspects of modern nursing, and have led us into a more dominant medical model of nursing care than ever before" (p. 937). Nurses also sustain this situation by wanting "to foster a professional, harder, rational, scientific and academic side" while maintaining the publicly held view of nursing as a *caring* profession. What is missing here from our perspective is the focus on nursing *qua* nursing, practiced as an expanded *human caring science.*

We argue that nursing's ethical, philosophical, and theoretical base can integrate caring and human phenomena within its disciplinary matrix, to become Caring Science, thus further differentiating nursing from medical science. Nursing scholars and theoretical discourses have demanded a shift to differentiate nursing from medicine, toward whole person expanded views of science for several decades. For example, Newman (1986, 1992), Newman, Sime, and Cororan-Perry (1991), Parse (1987, 1992), Rogers (1970, 1989), Sarter (1988), Watson (1979, 1988, 1995) all make a case for a different paradigm to differentiate nursing from medicine.

But even now it remains difficult to achieve due to competing dynamics and shifting priorities. Indeed, a recent Position paper on *Nursing Knowledge—Impact on Nursing's Preferred Future* from an Expert Panel of the American Academy of Nursing (Jones & Wright, 2010, pp. 2, 3) highlighted:

"The explosion of nursing theory in the . . . 1970s provided substance to the focus of the discipline, guided research and enhanced nursing's ability to articulate the substantive content of nursing and a professional vision. These works offered a worldview to guide knowledge development and expansion. . . . Nursing, described as a science and a human practice discipline, uses scientific knowledge and values to promote a caring relationship with patients, families and communities . . .".

However, within education, emphasis on integrating nursing knowledge into the educational preparation of nurses remains inconsistent.

Theory course are often taught in isolation, frequently abandoned throughout the curriculum as a whole; some disciplinary courses are being eliminated or changed to emphasize new roles. "More recently, the growth of the doctorate in nursing practice (DNP) (in its current iteration), minimizes the inclusion and translation of nursing theory. Other trends include developing nursing research and scholarship framed in other disciplines, which further compromises disciplinary knowledge development and advancement of the discipline and profession of nursing".

In light of the historic advancements and developments in the discipline, the current trends and detours, as noted in the AAN paper (2010), are troubling, and call forth another phase in nursing's disciplinary evolution. However, this next phase requires a transformative way of thinking. It calls for nurses to think about the discipline of nursing as an integration of artistry within an expanded view of science. Once one places the *human* and *caring* into a model of science, the model evolves, congruent with the timeless history, heritage, traditions, and practices of nursing.

Nursing's Ambivalent, Tormented Relationship With Medicine

Nursing has had, and continues to have, an ambivalent, tormented relationship with medicine. Nursing's current "angst," in this regard, must include sorting out and clarifying its relationship with medicine. Certainly, the two professions overlap (Figure 1.1). There is no question that nurses need medical knowledge in order to care for people, just as physicians need bedside caring manners to treat diseases. However, nursing and medicine are not the same.

Medicine's main focus is on diagnosing, treating, and curing diseases (Figure 1.2), whereas nursing's main focus is on caring for people and their experience of health-illness and healing (Figure 1.3).

Nursing and Medicine's knowledge and competencies overlap, yes, but the essence of what each profession does, and the knowledge base from within each, is quite different.

In addition to nurses having *medical* knowledge about disease processes, nurses also need *nursing* knowledge of caring and healing and the human health–illness experience. As a result, a nurse's domain of practice is precise: caring for the individual in relation to the individual's experience and meanings associated with health, recovery, and

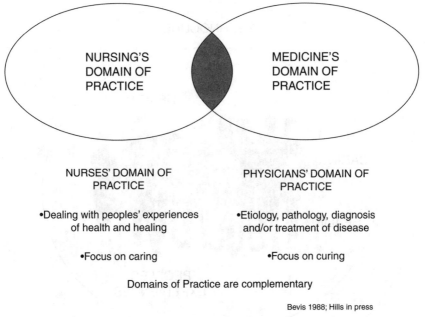

NURSES' DOMAIN OF
PRACTICE

•Dealing with peoples' experiences
of health and healing

•Focus on caring

PHYSICIANS' DOMAIN OF
PRACTICE

•Etiology, pathology, diagnosis
and/or treatment of disease

•Focus on curing

Domains of Practice are complementary

Bevis 1988; Hills in press

FIGURE 1.1   Complementary domains of practice.

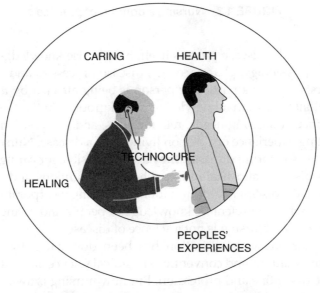

FIGURE 1.2   Medicine's domain of practice.

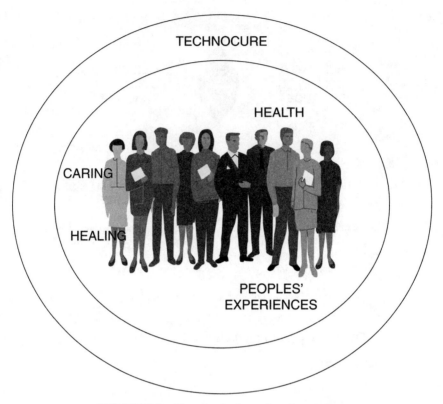

FIGURE 1.3 Nursing's domain of practice.

healing—not the disease process itself. Nurses use knowledge of anatomy and physiology, pharmacology, disease processes, and diagnosis to understand how a particular person is being affected by those processes. Nonetheless, that knowledge is background. In the foreground, there is focus on caring needs, relationships, and processes, the health and healing experience of a person living with a disease. Nurses are not responsible for curing diseases; they are responsible for caring for people with diseases and health-illness-healing conditions and concerns. As a result, the disciplinary foundation for nursing incorporates the ethics, philosophy, and scientific knowledge of people and caring–healing health practices. Nursing is not a science of diseases.

For years nursing education has been dominated by medical–clinical orientations and conventional medical science, *not* nursing as a complete discipline and profession. But now nursing is awakening to, and maturing within, its own human Caring Science foundation. As such, this awakening and this book reignite the caring curriculum, but now within a mature Caring Science context and enlightened views of caring pedagogies. It is not an either/or approach; it is a both/and approach to two complementary professions. Society needs the best of medicine and the best of nursing.

Now as the 21st century matures, nurse educators are invited anew to teach nursing as a more evolved discipline, based on a Caring Science curriculum, rather than a medically dominated focus.

Evidence-Based Practice

Nursing's current fascination with EBP is another example of how nursing continues to "follow" medicine rather than embrace its own science. The term "evidence-based nursing" evolved from the initial work done in evidence-based medicine, which was defined as "the conscientious explicit and judicious use of current best evidence in making decisions about the care of individual patients" (Sackett, Rosenberg, Gray, & Haynes, 1996, p. 71). In their landmark paper, the Evidence-based Medicine Working Group (1992) defined the primary source of evidence as randomized control trials (RCTs) and meta-analysis of RCTs. "Despite a later effort to partially ameliorate this definition, the original definition eventually grew into the hierarchy of levels of evidence that underpin the concept of evidence-based medicine" (Sackett et al., 1996). Here, the RCT remains the gold standard with an hierarchy of evidence entrenched in a positivist, reductionist ontology, epistemology, and methodology. Although this might work for medicine, many nursing scholars have recognized that the definitions of evidence espoused by the proponents of EBM are "too narrow and exclusive to support the complexities of nursing practice" (Estabrooks, 1998; Kitson, Harvey, & McCormack, 1998; Madjar & Walton, 2001; Rycroft-Malone et al., 2004; Tarlier, 2005). Furthermore, these hierarchy definitions of empiricism and objectivism as the dominant form of evidence, are incompatible with the complex and contextural knowledge of human health illness and human caring knowledge and processes (Palmer, 2004).

For nursing, several limitations and contradictions arise when attempting to adapt to an EBM approach to practice. First, if nursing is to claim the core of its domain of practice as Caring Science—with an expanded ethic, philosophy, and epistemology, focused on people and their experiences of health and healing—using an approach to EBP that is situated in a limited, reductionistic, positivist perspective is in conflict with, and antithetical to, the very essence of nursing and human caring processes. As Heron and Reason (1997) state:

> Orthodox research methods, as part of their rationale, exclude human subjects from all the thinking and decision making that generates and designs, manages and draws conclusions from the research. Such exclusions treat the subject as less than self-determining persons, alienates them from the inquiry process and from the knowledge that is its outcome, and thus invalidates any claim the methods have to a science of persons. (p. 280)

Further, an evidence-based approach tends to encourage nurses to overly focus on technical and technocure aspects in nursing; it is not oriented to include the more complex and sophisticated aspects of nursing's focus: people and inner meaning, perceptions, feelings, and the complex, relational, experiential, contextual aspects of health and healing. In fact, EBP, as conventionally designed, ignores caring as the moral and ethical practice of nursing and denies nursing's science of human caring. As Baumann (2010) suggests, "outcome-oriented EBP often fails to fully respect the primacy of the individual or to consider the importance of the meaning of the experience for the person" (p. 229).

Finally, nurses who base their practice exclusively on results from conventional evidence-based research through RCTs perhaps unknowingly reinforce the dichotomy of nursing—separating art from science, further compromising nursing's standing as a legitimate discipline and perpetuating nursing's ambivalent, tormented relationship with medicine.

For nursing to continue to evolve as a unique discipline, we need to critically examine our caring knowledge and practices and develop ways of revealing evidence that are consistent with the philosophical and theoretical foundation of a mature discipline and profession distinct from, but complementary to, medicine and all health professions.

WHAT IS CARING SCIENCE?
THE NEXT ENTRANCE AHEAD

For starters, "Caring Science can be defined as an evolving ethical-epistemic field of study that is grounded in the discipline of nursing and informed by related fields" (Watson & Smith, 2002, p. 456).

Throughout this book, we make Caring Science explicit as the disciplinary foundation of the nursing profession. In this chapter, we also explore the question, *What is Caring Science and why is it important in nursing education, practice and research?*

The *discipline* of nursing and the *profession* of nursing are not synonymous, and it is important for teachers and students alike to know and understand the difference between them. Understanding this difference is fundamental to designing and implementing a Caring Science curriculum.

The disciplinary foundation provides the moral and intellectual blueprint for education, practice, research, and leadership. It is the starting point for a professional orientation. More specifically, within the discipline of nursing are its knowledge and research traditions. The discipline offers the meta-narrative, worldview, historical heritage, theories, principles, assumptions, traditions, values, and the lens to view human and caring-healing-health phenomena. The discipline bridges the moral, philosophical, ethical, and theoretical foundations with practice demands and conventional expectations.

The disciplinary foundation guides the profession and the professional from the inside out, in contrast to outside in. Nonetheless, professional practice expectations and demands often result in the profession and the professional being whiplashed by the changing circumstances and external forces of our high-paced practice healthcare (sick care) system. Without disciplinary clarity, nursing can lose its way in the outer world of compromise and conformity, modeling itself on other developments (often originating from medical technology, industry, business and economics), rather than maturing as a distinct discipline in its own right. Witness the historical detours we have already noted in succumbing to outer forces: the dichotomy of art and science; the lingering, ambivalent relationship with medical science; and the limited approaches of EBP. Thus, we make explicit that there is a difference between nursing maturing within its own Caring Science paradigm and Nursing maturing within medicine's paradigm. The two paths exist but they are divergent.

Indeed, we can now acknowledge that as soon as nursing identifies its science as encompassing the *human* and the phenomena of *human caring* and *human health-illness experiences*—and their *meaning, relations,* and *context*—then we must make a case for a different model for nursing science, that is, Caring Science.

Incorporating caring and human experiences in a model of science demands a relational and ethical starting point and a relational worldview, which differs from medical science.

Caring Science provides this deep underpinning for a scientific-philosophical-moral context from which to explore, describe, and research human caring–healing phenomena as integral to our humanity. As the disciplinary foundation for nursing, Caring Science clarifies for the profession, and the professional, the question of ontology, that is, *what is our worldview of reality? What is the nature of Being and Becoming human in relation to the larger infinite universal field of life itself?*

Here, the starting point and underlying ontology is one of *relation* in contrast to *separation*. Caring Science does not separate mind from body, heart from head, person from environment-community, the human from the ecosystem. Caring Science also addresses a core question: what does it mean to be human? It acknowledges the unity of mindbodyspirit-environment-universe, as one entity; it makes explicit that we all *Belong* to the wider universal field of Planet Earth, the universe, the cosmos, the mystery, the void (Watson, 2005, 2008).

Caring Science helps us reflect upon what it means to be whole, to be healed, and to be caring. It reminds us—as we place, or re-place, human caring and the human experiences within a model of science—that we have a distinctive model of science that informs and inspires the discipline and profession of nursing; a model of science underpinned by a cosmology and ethic of unity, of belonging, of relations, of connectedness with the great circle, and of the web of life itself.

In terms of more concrete practicalities, Caring Science, ethically and philosophically, seeks to avoid reducing any human, whether student or patient or any other, to the moral status of object. For example, in the conventional world of daily nursing practice, a scenario, such as the following, can be quite common:

- Person is reduced to patient
- Patient is reduced to body physical
- Body physical is reduced to machine; thus, the human is reduced to the moral status of an object.

Once a human being has been reduced to the moral status of object, we professionals can separate ourselves from one another, can justify doing things to the *other*-as-*object* that we would never do to the other as a fully functioning human like ourselves (Watson, 2005, influenced by Gadow, previous personal communication). Furthermore, we know from humanity (including our own unique experiences) and the wisdom traditions across time that one person's level of humanity is reflected on another. If the person/patient is reduced to object status, then so is the nurse, the practitioner, and the teacher, even if she or he is not precisely aware of it. Therefore, it is the disciplinary lens, the values and the moral imperatives located within Caring Science philosophies and theories of nursing, which guide and sustain nursing in its covenant with humanity across time and space, worlds and change.

DISCIPLINARY FOUNDATION AS GUIDE TO ACTION

As teachers and students engage the consciousness of Caring Science, the moral-ethical-epistemic-spiritual dimensions of caring (and healing and humanity) become more explicit as a formal guide to action. Caring Science as a disciplinary foundation acknowledges

- a philosophy of human freedom, choice, responsibility, and human consciousness evolution;
- a biology and psychology of holism; a unity of *Being/Becoming*;
- an epistemology that allows not only for empirics, but also for the advancement of aesthetics, ethical values, intuition, personal-emotional knowing, spiritual insights, a process of discovery, creative imagination, joy, passion, and evolving forms of inquiry;
- an ontology of time and space;
- a context of inter-subjective human experiences, events, processes, and relationships that connect with/are at-one-with the environment and the wider universe; and
- a scientific worldview that is open, guided by ethics as first principle and starting point for humans and Being-in-the-world (Levinas, 1969; Watson, 1985, p. 16; Watson, 2008);
- Caring Knowledge is, as a serious epistemic endeavor, not to be assumed or taken for granted.

A Caring Science orientation differs from conventional science and invites qualitatively different aspects of our shared humanity in the universe that are to be honored as legitimate and necessary. This is especially true when working with humanity, human experiences, human caring–healing, life phenomena, and all the vicissitudes of human living:

> Facing ourself and our humanity . . .
> Is a moral act
> And comes before clinical knowledge;
> . . . the value-laden human condition . . .
> Vulnerability, pain, suffering and discomfort,
> Are value-laden phenomena;
> They are moral realities

(Nortvedt, 2000, p. 2, in Watson, 2005, p. 44)

It is imperative to be explicit about one's starting point and core values, since one's moral-ethical starting point determines where one ends up. For example, if one starts with a professional, clinical-medical lens regarding humanity and one's phenomena of focus, then that medical professional lens guides one's approach to teaching, learning, and practicing nursing.

If we start with a disciplinary lens in Caring Science that values, honors and acknowledges the wholeness of humanity, our oneness with each other and all aspects of humanity, and our place in the wider universe, then we can be open to unknowns and the fullness of our humanity, dwelling in paradox, ambiguity, mystery, and even miracles. The overall Caring Science disciplinary lens allows for our own and others' evolution and for transformation of consciousness. Thus, personal growth, change, insight, humility, spirit-guided inner resources, and wisdom are present in the moment in human-to-human caring relationships. This allows for *caring moments* to occur between student-teacher or between nurse-patient. The disciplinary foundation helps the nursing profession to sustain and enact its deep values, its *raison d'etre* in the world, and its commitment to humanity itself. As one of our colleagues in England put it

> Any profession which loses its values becomes Heartless;
> Any professional which becomes heartless, becomes Soulless;
> Any profession that becomes heartless and soulless becomes Worthless!

(Eagger, 2001, personal communication)

Again, Caring Science differs from conventional science in several significant ways as identified in Table 1.1.

TABLE 1.1   Differences Between Conventional and Caring Science

CONVENTIONAL SCIENCE	CARING SCIENCE
ONTOLOGY: Worldview	ONTOLOGY AS ETHIC
Neutrality of Values	Ethic/ontology of Belonging as first principle
Paternalistic–External Control	
A separatist worldview as starting point	Connectedness, Interdependence; Inner control
A stance toward clinical distance, separation, control—attempt to be neutral or value free with objective assumptions	A relational unitary worldview as starting point
	Values: preserving humanity, human caring, dignity, human spirit, wholeness, integrity, unity
EPISTEMOLOGICAL RESTRICTIONS	EPISTEMOLOGICAL PLURALISM
Limited Epistemology Knowledge: Objective–factual procedural, outer knowledge—empirics as starting point; reductionistic epistemology	Expanded epistemology
	Honoring all ways of Knowing/Being/Becoming; diversity of knowledge development, cocreated from inside out and outside in; move from information to knowledge to understanding to meaning to wisdom to inner knowing. Multiple forms of "evidence" from empirics to aesthetic, noetic, poetic, personal, intuitive, ethical, mystical and even spiritual knowing . . . allowing for "elegance, beauty, simplicity and parsimony as alternative theoretical-scientific explanatory models" (Watson, 2005, p. 28).
METHODOLOGY	CARING INQUIRY
Experimental scientifically controlled research methods; largely quantitative objective data is what counts as "evidence," as knowledge	Caring Science Methodology allows for multiple forms of "evidence" and diverse methods, forms of inquiry, open to creative-artistic-visionary, narrative, performance, expanded epistemological approaches to research and knowledge development, while incorporating empirical data
PRACTICE	PRAXIS
Professional scientific, clinicalized–medicalized views of humanity and human conditions; efforts to "fix the parts," control human processes and environment, treat disease and body physical (often at all costs) from external treatments mechanisms; outer curing focus	Practice shifts to *praxis*—that is, reflective practice informed by disciplinary foundational values, theories, philosophical-ethical stance; informed by meaning, context, relations, and knowledgeable caring-healing practices; honoring deeply spirit-filled dimensions of humankind

We can see from Table 1.1 that a Caring Science *disciplinary* starting point informs and guides our approach to given phenomena. It is important for us to clarify our disciplinary starting point to make explicit the focus and direction of nursing education, of a caring curriculum, of approaches to knowledge development, of learning-teaching, of teaching strategies, and of pedagogy. In turn, our entire intellectual consciousness of Caring Science informs our professional practices and development of the profession itself. This consciousness affects our approaches to self-knowledge and to humanity in general.

A Caring Science curriculum provides the disciplinary map for teaching-learning nursing. It may be in contrast to, or even in conflict with, conventional nursing models and blueprints of education and practice that are guided by a historical, medicalized, technical, or more established professional focus.

What Is a Caring Science Curriculum?

> It is time for the nursing educational system to question the impact our current curricular and pedagogical approaches might be having on nurses' ability to work effectively beyond the demand for technical competence at the bedside; nurses need to be politically active, work autonomously, and create the sort of caring-healing practices that first attracted most nurses into the profession.
>
> Clark (2002, p. 25, in Clark, 2010, p. 42)

A Caring Science curriculum lays a solid foundation for reconnecting the heart, soul, mind, emotions, and the human spirit of students and teachers alike; it invites passion, intellect, moral ideals, and love into our classrooms and curriculum, restoring humanity and human caring-healing knowledge and practices for now and the future. Danish philosopher Logstrup helps make explicit that educators, quite literally and metaphorically, hold other people's lives in their hands.

> By our value/attitude to the other person, we help to determine the scope and hue of his/her world; we make it larger or smaller, bright or drab, rich or dull, threatening or secure.
>
> We help to shape his/her world, not by theories and views but by our very being and attitude toward other.
>
> Herein lies the unarticulated and, one might say, anonymous demand that we take care of life which trust has placed in our hands. (Logstrup, 1997, p. 18)

CORE INGREDIENTS OF A CARING SCIENCE CURRICULUM

A Caring Science curriculum seeks to create authentic, egalitarian, human-to-human relationships. This assumption is based on the notion that there is reciprocity between power, knowledge, and control, and that, in order for there to be more equitable relationships, those with power need to give up and share control, so that others may benefit and share their knowledge, thus their power. Authentic power is shared power; it is power with, not power over. It does not negate faculty or nurses' responsibilities, skills or knowledge. It also means standing in one's own power, one's own truth and integrity, without succumbing to other's position of power, authoritarian control, and so on.

We can still acknowledge the reality that there is a difference between having authority and being authoritarian; the teacher has authority by the nature of her/his position; however, that does not justify an authoritarian, power-control stance toward knowledge, toward students, and toward control of knowledge. In a Caring Science curriculum, students also have authority in their own knowing and experiences that can be shared and jointly critiqued for deeper knowledge, understanding, integrative insights and wisdom, ultimately, resulting in transformation of consciousness.

To create such a visionary Caring Science curriculum for human caring–healing, Noddings (1984) has identified at least four ingredients of a caring curriculum that flow from Caring Science as the starting point. They are

- Modeling—not role modeling in the sense of modeling after someone else; rather assisting others to model their best self;
- Practice—living day-to-day experiences in the living relationships between and among students and faculty, and between and among students, in and out of the classroom, virtual settings, and clinical setting—creating a community of caring environment that holds the entire program;
- Authentic dialogue—in keeping with the realization that imparting knowledge is not learning, a caring curriculum creates space for students to have authentic dialogue, allowing questions and discussions, exploration of ideas and knowledge to comingle for new insights, process discovery, and transformation of consciousness;

- Confirmation—or Affirmation—This philosophical perspective guides the educator to hold the student in their highest ethical ideal of self, even if the student cannot see that ideal for themselves in the moment. (This notion transfers into the clinical setting, whereby a Caring Science practitioner holds the patient in their wholeness, even if the patient is experiencing pain and illness.)

These four ingredients are philosophical and ethical, as well as practical orientations to hold in our framework for implementing and living out a Caring Science curriculum. These ingredients flow from underlying beliefs and values that can be made explicit in a Caring Science context.

Once we are clear about the disciplinary direction for nursing, then curricular issues and directions become more consistent; we are less compromised by conventional mind-sets and the status quo. We are less tied to or caught up within previously established, limiting approaches to education, to teaching-learning, and to traditional pedagogical issues. A new horizon of moral ideals, inspiration, creativity, human spirit, liberation, intellectual passion, joy, and even spiritual freedom is available to all.

Time Out for Reflection

How would you define a Caring Science curriculum?

What does Caring Science offer for nursing education and practice?

What is the difference between the discipline of nursing and the profession of nursing? Why is this difference important to understand?

What are the factors that distinguish a Caring Science curriculum from another type of nursing curriculum?

EVOLUTION OF CURRICULUM DIRECTIONS: CURRENT DILEMMAS

Nurse educators continue to face challenges in addressing curriculum reform from nursing's disciplinary foundation. For example, recent AACN national reports (i.e., White paper on the education and role of the Clinical Nurse Leader; the essentials of doctoral education for advanced nursing practice; the essentials of baccalaureate education for professional nursing practice, AACN, 2006, 2007, 2008) have been critiqued as having *insufficient emphasis . . .* on the *disciplinary knowledge of nursing...*" (Smith & McCarthy, 2010, p. 44). This gap between educational recommendations and the need for disciplinary knowledge as foundation makes it all the more important that we in nursing education, and scholars of nursing education, review and critique such documents and reports for their strengths and shortcomings. As part of nursing maturing as a health and caring profession, distinct from, but complementary to, medicine, it is important that major educational blueprints are critiqued within the most contemporary scholarly discourse. Thus, the work of creating a Caring Science curriculum requires nursing educators and progressive educational programs and curricula to acknowledge, benefit from, and critique current reports and documents, to incorporate the most current scholarly discourse of nursing.

As noted in the recent American Academy of Nursing Expert Panel paper (2010, p. 2) "Nursing theories, developed by Academy leaders . . . and many others, have provided the discipline with innovative worldviews to guide practice, affect and sustain behavior change and enhance understanding of the human condition. **These approaches provide strategies to help providers move away from the prescriptive . . . 'this is what you should do' strategies . . .**" (Our emphasis).

A Caring Science curriculum seeks to move beyond conventional blueprints and relocate all generalist and advanced specialist nursing education within the philosophies, ethics, theories, research, and practice models that originate from the disciplinary foundation of nursing.

Indeed, our challenge and request is that you, as nurse educators, critique these, and any other documents, explore educational scholarship that ensures that our future nurses will be prepared, educated, informed, inspired, and passionate about nursing maturing as a Caring Science. By doing so, you help to assure that the disciplinary ground is established to distinguish and guide education, practices and research in nursing (*qua* nursing) for future generations.

Traditionally, curriculum has been thought of as a planned program of studies or a blueprint for learning, focusing largely on content and dissemination of objective clinical data, information, procedural knowledge for technological competencies, and skills. Important as these dimensions are, a Caring Science orientation to curriculum takes a marked shift from those past, conventional, views. As Bevis and Watson (1989, 2000) explained, conventional nursing educators have typically shuffled content around within the curriculum structure declaring this *swapping and switching* as *curriculum change*, when no real change has actually taken place.

Despite the shortcoming and critiques of the aforementioned documents and reports, and while we are inviting still another evolutionary turn, it is important to acknowledge that curricular changes have occurred in nursing education over the past decade or so toward more humane and humanitarian approaches to teaching, learning, and practice.

At least in part, these changes have occurred due to the National League for Nursing's *caring curriculum revolution* series of programs, publications, and conferences held during the 1980s, and were further influenced by Bevis and Watson's (1989) redefinition of curriculum as "the interactions and transactions that occur between and among teachers and students in order that learning occur" (p. 6), with curriculum linked more than ever to a view of the person as whole. As Bevis and Watson indicated, the teacher's pedagogical skills encompassed student-faculty learning relationships and sought inspired teaching-learning within the context of these relationships. This reorientation to the relationship between and among teachers and students, and teachers' pedagogical skills has had a tremendous impact on the teaching of nursing over the last 20 plus years.

Of course, pedagogy is discussed at length in later chapters. We agree here, that it is the heart of curriculum development and the space that invites learning. In the meantime, we can point to inspired pedagogical changes that have spilled over from the curriculum revolution and which represent the heart of curriculum change.

Progressive nurse educators responded to pedagogical challenges identified by the curriculum revolutionaries, and, as a result, we see hopeful current changes in relational learning; a renewed interest in active learning; student-centered learning (Diekelmann, 2004; Young & Paterson, 2007); interactive learning, context-based learning (Williams & Day, 2007); story-based learning (Young, 2007); narrative pedagogy (Diekelmann, 2005; Brown & Rodney, 2007); and transformative virtual pedagogy (Watson, 2002).

Although these developments represent important progress in articulating innovative *pedagogical* approaches for nursing education, only a few authors (Giddens & Brady, 2007; Hills & Lindsey, 1994; Iwasiw et al., 2005; Jillings & O'Flynn-Magee, 2007) along with Boykin & Schoenhofer, 2001; Mary Enzman Hines, 2011; Mary Rockwood Lane, 2011; and Sitzman, 2007 (see chapters in this text) have attempted to outline different approaches to the *structure and organizational aspects of curriculum development*. All of these historic and contemporary trends and turns in nursing education are evolutionary in the sense that they each contribute to a new dimension in curriculum thinking and pedagogical processes. However, there is still another turn to be made that underpins these curricular processes and structures.

For example, other, earlier reports from national professional organizations and educational foundations reflect the authentic, evolutionary spiral still needed. The 1994 Pew-Fetzer Task Group Report on Relationship-Centered Care for all health professions, the New Essentials of Nursing Education: BS, MS, DNS document of the American Association of Colleges of Nursing [AACN] (2009), and the early Boyer report (1990) addressed the need for serious reform. This need was highlighted again in the more recent Carnegie Report on Nursing Education, by Benner, Sutphen, Leonard, and Day (2010). This Carnegie report specifically recommended dramatic changes in how nurses are educated: "immersing nursing students in the *discipline* (our italics) of nursing during the first two years of study" (2010). Each of these reports in some way critiques the status quo for nursing and health science professional education and makes a case for caring relationships and foundational basics as the essential core of educational reform.

Although many nursing educators today seek to embrace expanded views of professional education and curriculum, nursing education on the whole has yet to actualize this broader vision proposed by earlier and more recent reports and recommendations. Indeed, in the recent publication by Caring Science scholars Smith and McCarthy (2010), faculty are encouraged to "go beyond these earlier and recent blueprints to educate generalist, advanced generalist, and advanced specialty nurses who are grounded in the philosophies, theories, research and practice models within the *discipline* (our italics) of nursing" (p. 44). Still, despite reports, recommendations and specific changes to make the necessary shift from **teaching** knowledge, techniques, procedures, and content toward authentic disciplinary **learning** (between and among faculty and students), there remains a gap between the status quo and creating a caring curriculum and one that is explicitly based within its most mature, evolved disciplinary foundation—in this instance: Caring Science.

There are notable exceptions, especially the curriculum work of Lewis and Naef (2006), who describe their efforts at York University, Ontario, Canada, within a human science/caring paradigm. Their work is guided by an explicit focus on human/Caring Science, which is evolutionary in itself, moving, as it has, beyond the Bevis and Watson text that emphasized the educative paradigm of critical thinking and critical social theory. Their work is described in a later contributed chapter. Dr. Anne Boykin, with her visionary, sustained Caring Science leadership and successes with her colleagues and the college-wide programs at Florida Atlantic University, is another noteworthy exception. They have also contributed a chapter to this book. The University of Victoria in Canada is a third example in which a collaborative curriculum was based on a philosophy of caring and health promotion. You will find this program discussed in Chapter 8 to highlight different frameworks and processes for curriculum development. These current successful programs and projects serve as hopeful models and exemplars of movement toward a mature Caring Science educational model for nursing.

NEXT TURN IN CURRICULUM EVOLUTION

The need remains to move more explicitly toward a curriculum that is grounded in, and builds upon, Caring Science as a more evolved disciplinary guide for structural organization, content, context, pedagogical strategies, and meaningful relationships. For now and the near future, the requirement is to prepare nurses as mature caring-healing-health practitioners of nursing, informed by their distinct discipline.

In this book, we offer a guide to creating a nursing curriculum that is grounded in the disciplinary matrix of Caring Science, going beyond the conventional blueprints, offering a model that serves as an emancipatory, even passionate, ethical-philosophical, educational and pedagogical learning guide for both teachers and students, and the caring relationship for both teaching and learning. The next chapter moves us further into this territory.

REFERENCES

American Association of Colleges of Nursing. (2007). *White paper on the education and role of the clinical nurse leader.* Washington, DC: Author.

American Association of Colleges of Nursing. (2008). *The essentials of baccalaureate education for professional nursing practice.* Washington, DC: Author.

American Association of Colleges of Nursing. (2009). *The essentials of doctoral education for advanced nursing practice.* Washington, DC: Author.

Baumann, S. (2010). The limitations of evidence-based practice. *Nursing Science Quarterly, 23*(93), 226–230.

Benner, P., Sutphen, M., Leonard, V., & Day, L. (2010). *Educating nurses: A call for radical transformation. The carnegie report for the advancement of teaching.* San Francisco: Jossey-Bass.

Bevis, E. O. (1988). *Curriculum building in nursing. A process* (3rd ed.). New York: NLN.

Bevis, E. O., & Watson, J. (1989). *Toward a caring curriculum. A new pedagogy for nursing.* New York: NLN.

Bevis, E. O., & Watson, J. (2000). *Towards a caring curriculum: A new pedagogy for nursing.* London: Jones & Bartlett.

Boyer, E. (1990). *Scholarship reconsidered: Priorities for the professoriate.* Princeton, NJ: Carnegie Foundation for the Advancement of Teaching.

Boykin, A., & Schoenhofer, S. (2001). *Nursing as caring: A model for transforming practice.* London: Jones & Bartlett Publishers.

Brown, H., & Rodney, P. (2007). In L. Young & B. Paterson (Eds.), *Teaching nursing: Developing a student-centered learning environment.* Philadelphia: Lippincott Williams & Wilkins.

Castledine, G. (2010). Creative nursing: Art or science? *British Journal of Nursing, 19,* 937–938.

Clark, C. S. (2010). The nursing shortage as a community transformational opportunity. *Advances in Nursing Science, 33*(1), 35–52.

Cowling, W. R., Smith, M. C., & Watson, J. (2008). The power of wholeness, consciousness and caring. A dialogue on nursing science, art, and healing. *Advances in Nursing Science, 31,* E41–E51.

Diekelmann, N. (2004). Class evaluations: Creating new student partnerships in support of innovation. *Journal of Nursing Education, 43*(10), 436–439.

Diekelmann, N. (2005). Engaging the students and the teacher: Co-creating substantive reform with narrative pedagogy. *Journal of Nursing Education, 44*(6), 249–252.

Eagger, S. (2001). Personal communication. In J. Watson (Ed.), *Caring science as sacred science.* Philadelphia: FA Davis.

Elfrink, V., & Lutz, E. (2009). *American Association of Colleges of Nursing essential values: National study of faculty perceptions, practices, and plans.* Washington, DC: Author.

Estabrooks, C. (1998). Will evidence-based nursing practice make practice perfect? *Canadian Journal of Nursing Research, 30,* 15–36.

Fawcett, J., Watson, J., Neuman, B., Walker, P., & Fitzpatrick, J. (2001). On nursing theories and evidence. *Journal of Nursing Scholarship, 33,* 115–119.

Freshwater, D. (2004). Aesthetics and evidence-based practice in nursing: An oxymoron? *International Journal of Human Caring* (serial online), *8,* 8–12.

Giddens, J., & Brady, D. (2007). Rescuing nursing education from content saturation: The case for a concept-based curriculum. *Journal of Nursing Education, 46*(2), 65–70.

Heron, J., & Reason, P. (1997). A participatory inquiry paradigm. *Qualitative Inquiry, 3*(3), 274–294.

Hills, M., & Lindsey, E. (1994). Health promotion: A viable framework for nursing education. *Nursing Outlook, 42*(4), 465–462.

Iwasiw, C., Goldenberg, D., & Andrusyszyn, M. (2008). *Curriculum development in nursing education.* Boston: Jones & Bartlett Publishers.

Jones, D., & Wright, B. (2010). *Nursing knowledge—Impact on nursing's preferred future. Position paper: Expert panel on nursing theory-guided practice.* American Academy of Nursing (submitted).

Jillings, C., & O'Flynn-Magee, K. (2007). Barriers to student-centered teaching: Overcoming institution and attitudinal obstacles. In L. Young & B. Paterson (Eds.), *Teaching nursing: Developing a student-centered learning environment* (pp. 467–483). Philadelphia: Lippincott Williams & Wilkins.

Kitson, A., Harvey, G., & McCormack, B. (1998). Enabling the implementation of evidence-based practice: A conceptual framework. *Quality in Health Care, 7,* 149–158.

Levinas, E. (1969). *Totality and infinity.* Pittsburgh, PA: Duquesne University.

Lewis, R., & Naef, M. R. (2006). Caring-human science philosophy in nursing education: Beyond the curriculum revolution. *International Journal of Human Caring, 10*(4), 31–37.

Logstrup, K. (1997). *The ethical demand.* Notre Dame, IN: University of Notre Dame.

Madjar, I., & Walton, J. (2001). What is problematic about evidence? In J. Morse, J. Swanson, & A. Kuzel (Eds.), *The nature of qualitative evidence* (pp. 28–45). Thousand Oaks, CA: Sage.

Moccia, P. (1988). *Curriculum revolution: An agenda for change. In curriculum revolution. mandate for change.* New York: NLN.

Munhall, P. (1981). Nursing philosophy and nursing research: In apposition or opposition? *Nursing Research, 31*(3), 176–181.

Munhall, P. (1988). *Curriculum revolution: A social mandate for change. In curriculum revolution: Mandate for change.* New York: NLN.

Newman, M. A. (1986). *Health as expanding consciousness.* St. Louis, MO: Mosby.

Newman, M. A. (1992). Prevailing paradigms in nursing. *Nursing Outlook, 40*(1), 10–13.

Newman, M. A., Sime, A. M., & Cororan-Perry, S. A. (1991). The focus of the discipline of nursing. *Advances in Nursing Science, 14*(1), 1–6.

Newman, M. A., Smith, M. C., Pharris, M. C., & Jones, D. (2008). The focus of the discipline revisite. *Advances in Nursing Science, 8*(31), E16–E27.

Nightingale, F. (1860). *Notes on nursing: What it is, and what it is not.* New York: Appleton.

Noddings, N. (1984). *Caring: A feminine approach to ethics and moral education.* Berkeley, CA: University of California Press.

Nortvedt, P. (2000). Clinical sensitivity: The inseparability of ethical perceptiveness and clinical knowledge. *Scholarly Inquiry for Nursing Practice, 14*(3), 1–19.

Palmer, P. (2004). *The violence of our knowledge. Toward a spirituality of higher education. 21st learning initiative.* Kalamazoo, MI: Fetzer Institute.

Parse, R. R. (1987). *Nursing science: Major paradigm, theories and critiques.* Philadelphia: Saunders.

Parse, R. R. (1992). Human becoming: Parse's theory of nursing. *Nursing Science Quarterly, 5,* 35–32.

Rogers, M. E. (1970). *An introduction to the theoretical basis of nursing.* Philadelphia: Davis.

Rogers, M. E. (1989). Nursing: A science of unitary human beings. In J. Riehl-Sisca (Ed.), *Conceptual models for nursing practice* (pp. 181–188). Englewood Cliffs, NJ: Appleton and Lange.

Rycroft-Malone, J., Seers, K., Titchen, A., Harvey, G., Kitson, A., & Mc Cormack, B. (2004). What counts as evidence in evidence-based practice? *Journal of Advanced Nursing, 47,* 81–90.

Sackett, D., Rosenberg, W., Gray, J., & Haynes, R. (1996). Evidence-based medicine: What it is and what it isn't. *British Medical Journal, 312,* 71–72.

Sarter, B. (1988). Philosophical sources of nursing theory. *Nursing Science Quarterly, 1,* 52–59.

Smith, H. (1982). *Beyond the postmodern mind.* New York: Crossroads Publications.

Smith, L. (1993). The art and science of nursing. *Nursing Times, 89*(25), 42–43.

Smith, M., & McCarthy, P. (2010). Disciplinary knowledge in nursing education: Going beyond the blueprints. *Nursing Outlook, 58,* 44–51.

Sitzman, K. L. (2007). Teaching-learning professional caring based on Jean Watson's theory of human caring. *International Association of Human Caring, 11*(4), 8–16.

Tanner, C. (1988). *Curriculum revolution: The practice mandate.* New York: NLN.

Tarlier, D. (2005). Mediating the meaning of evidence through epistemological diversity. *Nursing Inquiry, 12(2),* 126–134.

Tresolini, C., & Pew-Fetzer Task Group. (1994). *Health professions education and relationship-centered care. Report of the Pew-Fetzer task force on advancing psychological health education.* San Francisco: Pew Health Professions Commission.

Watson, J. (1979). *Nursing the philosophy and science of caring.* Boston: Little Brown.

Watson, J. (1985, 2007). *Nursing: Human science and human care.* Boston: Jones and Bartlett. (Connecticut, USA: Appleton-Century-Crofts Reprinted 2007).

Watson, J. (1988). New dimensions of human caring theory. *Nursing Science Quarterly, 1,* 175–181.

Watson, J. (1995). Postmodern knowledge development in nursing. *Nursing Science Quarterly, 8*(2), 60–64.

Watson, J. (2002). Metaphysics of virtual caring communities. *International Journal of Human Caring, 6*(1), 41–45.

Watson, J. (2005). *Caring science as sacred science.* Philadelphia: FA Davis.

Watson, J. (2008). *Nursing: The philosophy and science of caring* (Rev. ed.). Boulder, CO: University Press of Colorado.

Watson, J., & Smith, M. (2002). Caring science and the science of unitary human beings. A transtheoretical discourse. *Journal of Advanced Nursing, 37*(5), 452–461.

Williams, B., & Day, R. (2007). Context-based learning. In L. Young & B. Paterson (Eds.), *Teaching nursing: Developing a student-centered learning environment.* Philadelphia: Lippincott Williams & Wilkins.

Willis, D. G., Grace, P. J., & Roy, C. (2008). A central unifying focus for the discipline: Facilitating humanization, meaning, choice, quality of life and healing our living and dying. *Advances in Nursing Science, 31,* E28–E40.

Young, L. (2007). Story-based learning: Blending content and process to learn nursing. In L. Young & B. Paterson (Eds.), *Teaching nursing: Developing a student-centered learning environment.* Philadelphia: Lippincott Williams & Wilkins.

Young, L., & Paterson, B. (Eds.). (2007). *Teaching nursing: Developing a student-centered learning environment.* Philadelphia: Lippincott Williams & Wilkins.

2

Beliefs and Assumptions: The Hidden Drivers of Curriculum Development

. . . a philosophical belief in human freedom—a "Wide
Awakeness" that is paradigm shattering and emancipatory . . .
calls for encouragement, self-reflection . . . educators come
in touch with their own humanity . . . encourage the release
of the human spirit . . .
—From Maxine Greene (1978) cited in Jean Watson (1989, p. 37)

T HE PURPOSE OF THIS CHAPTER is to highlight the important role
that beliefs, values, and assumptions play in guiding our thinking, behavior, and actions in general, as we engage in the curriculum development process, and, specifically, the influence they have
on our pedagogical practices, ultimately student–teacher relationships
and knowing. We address the underlying beliefs and assumptions
of a Caring Science curriculum in order to help faculty and students
gain clarity about just what Caring Science is and why, we argue, it
must form the foundation of the *discipline* of Nursing. This foundation of beliefs and assumptions opens up the heart and mind to the
beauty and manifestation of Caring Science as a serious and emancipatory epistemic, ethical, ontological, pedagogical, methodological, and
praxis endeavor.

IMPACT OF BELIEFS ON WORLD VIEW AND BEHAVIOR

Beliefs and assumptions are embedded in and deeply influence our
worldview, our perceptions, and our actions in everyday experiences.
It is important to be aware of our beliefs and assumptions because they

influence our thinking, our learning, and our ways of interacting as we encounter experiences. In fact, they determine the meaning that we give a specific situation at any moment in time; they reflect our level of consciousness and our own evolution, which in turn affects our very view of reality.

Our beliefs are convictions that we hold as "truths." They may not actually be true but, within ourselves, they are the "facts" that we hold as "Truth." For example, we may believe that "we cannot teach anyone anything." This may not be "true" but, because it is a belief we hold, we will act as if it were true. We all have many beliefs, and, although they may change from time to time, many of us operate in the world unaware of the beliefs we hold. Many of these beliefs may have been with us since childhood and may, in fact, no longer be relevant to one's current circumstances and context. For example, we may unconsciously hold the belief "people can't be trusted"; thus, this embedded belief from childhood will affect our interactions and ability to relate to others. We also have many conflicting beliefs and, at times, may have difficulty making decisions because of these conflicting beliefs.

Although our beliefs have an epistemic status (i.e., they make assumptions about what is "true"), often they are more deeply embedded in and determined by our "values," or those things we attach worth to. This makes some of our beliefs difficult to change and even highly resistant to change. Egan (1985) suggests that if you want to understand what your values are, you should monitor how you spend your time. For example, he suggests that if you say that you value reading but when asked when was the last time that you read a book, you respond that you don't have time to read, he would say that reading is not a value for you. Similarly, if you say that you value patient-centered care but you say that you don't have time to talk to your patients because there is too much to do, your behavior does not support your stated values. So, think about how you spend your time. Combs (1982) describes this process as learning to read behavior backwards.

The most important idea to take away from this discussion about beliefs and assumptions is to appreciate how these fundamental aspects of human nature affect your behavior, your consciousness, and in turn your very worldview, particularly in relation to curriculum development and pedagogical situations.

To demonstrate this point, we share this story that Combs (1979) shared when talking to a group of educators. Consider your experiences with teaching/learning situations as you read the story.

In a school in the outskirts of Atlanta there was a young woman teaching the first grade who was a very beautiful young woman with a beautiful head of blonde hair that she was accustomed to wearing in a pony tail that hung down to the middle of her back. The first few days of school she wore her hair this way. Then on Thursday, she decided she wanted to do it differently, so she did it all up in a bun on the top of her head. One of the little boys in her class looked into her room but he didn't recognize his teacher, you know that happens sometimes when a woman changes her hairdo, because she doesn't look like the same person. So here he was, lost and the bell rang and school started and he didn't know where to go. Along came the supervisor and found this little boy in the hall crying and she said to him, "What is the trouble?" and he said, "I can't find my teacher." So she said, "What is your teacher's name?" And he didn't know, so she said, "What room are you in?" and he didn't know that either. He had looked in there and it was the wrong place. So she said, "Well come on. Let's see if we can find her." And they started down the hall opening one door after another without much luck. Finally, they came to the room where this young woman was teaching and she opened the door and she saw the supervisor and the little boy and she said, "Why Joey, it is so good to see you. We have been wondering where you were. Come on in. We have missed you so." And the little boy pulled out of the supervisor's hand and threw himself into the teacher's arms. She gave him a hug and patted him on the fanny and he ran down to his seat. Now the supervisor was telling me this story and said to me, "You know, I said a prayer for that teacher. She thought little boys were important."

As the supervisor was telling me this story we were riding along in a car. We got to playing a game, you know. We said, "Well suppose she hadn't thought that little boys were important." Suppose for instance, she thought supervisors were important. Well in that case she might have said, "Why, good morning Miss Cheeves. We have been hoping that you would come by and see us, haven't we boys and girls?" Or she might have thought that discipline was important. And in that case she might have said, "Joey you know very well when you are late you must go to the office and get a permit, now run right down there." Or she might have thought the lesson was important. In that case she might have said, "Joey, for heaven's sake where have you been, get your books and get to work." But she didn't, she thought that little boys were important and she behaved in terms of what she thought was important. So it is with all of us. We are discovering that this is what makes the difference between a good counsellor and a poor one, or a good teacher and a poor one, or a good nurse and a poor one or a good priest and a poor one.

What do you believe is important?

This story provides an excellent illustration of how our beliefs, values, and assumptions are apparent in our behavior, affecting our consciousness, our worldview, and our response to any given situation.

LEARNING ACTIVITY:
ACTIONS SPEAK LOUDER THAN WORDS

Ends in View

The purpose of this learning activity is to become aware of how our beliefs, values, and assumptions are present in our behaviors.

In your journal, divide the page by drawing a line down the middle of it. In the left-hand column, write five beliefs that you have that are consistent with a Caring Science curriculum. In the right-hand column, write a corresponding action that you take that demonstrates that belief or value. Over the next week, monitor your behaviors; your awareness of your thoughts and state of our consciousness and views toward any given situation. Reflect in your journal about what beliefs and values seem evident to you based on your behaviors and evolving consciousness related to beliefs and values.

Time Out for Reflection

Reflect on your beliefs, values, and corresponding actions.

Share your reflections with your learning partner or group.

Consider the following questions:

Did you have similar beliefs or values but different actions?

Was the relationship between your beliefs or values and your actions apparent?

What is your understanding of the relationship between your beliefs or values and your actions?

Becoming aware of your beliefs and assumptions, particularly in relation to how they "show up" in your behavior, can prove to be a very insightful exercise. Many of us behave without really being aware of what is driving our behavior, not being aware of how we "see the world" through our own value lens.

Learning to monitor your beliefs and assumptions will assist you in discarding those that are no longer relevant or that don't fit with your desire to develop a Caring Science worldview. Such a shift in beliefs and assumptions reflects a change in, or evolution of consciousness, affecting your very view of the world.

Learning to do so will assist you in becoming a much more critically reflective practitioner and teacher. For example, one definition of "theory" goes back to the Latin word "theoria," which literally means "to see"; as we engage in this simple exercise, we find new lenses "to see" our reality in new ways. When one can critique one's own beliefs and "see" things differently, then one can act differently (Watson, 2008a).

The following is a synopsis of a fascinating study conducted a number of years ago. Combs (1971) examined the factors that influence a teacher's effectiveness. He was interested in knowing what the differences were between effective and ineffective teachers. At first, he thought it might be the knowledge that teachers had about a certain subject, but he discovered that knowledge was not a critical factor in teacher effectiveness. As you may have experienced, many teachers are knowledgeable about their subject matter but are not effective teachers! In this initial work, he also discovered that the methods teachers used did not influence their effectiveness, nor did their theoretical perspectives.

Teachers who were considered to be effective were more like one another than like other teachers who practiced from similar theoretical perspectives but were less effective. As he pursued his research, he *discovered that it wasn't the knowledge, methods or theoretical perspective that made a teacher effective but rather the nature of the interaction and the beliefs that teachers held that were of paramount importance in determining teaching effectiveness* (our emphasis). Combs tested 12 hypotheses in 5 different areas regarding the beliefs held by teachers that made them effective or not effective. These are summarized below (Table 2.1).

TABLE 2.1   Differences Between Effective and Ineffective Teachers

EFFECTIVE TEACHERS	INEFFECTIVE TEACHERS
Beliefs About Frame of Reference	
• Other Oriented	• Self-Oriented
• Focus on People	• Focus on Things—rules, regulations, test results
Beliefs About People	
• People are Able—they have the capacity to handle their own problems	• People are not Able—would be unethical to let someone do something if you didn't believe they were able to do it
• People are Friendly	• People are Basically Unfriendly
• People are Worthy of Dignity and Integrity	• People are Unworthy of Dignity and Integrity
• People are Dependable	• People are Not Dependable
Beliefs About Self	
• Identify with Others	• Feel Apart (Different) from Others
• Feel They are "Enough" the Way They are	• Feel They are Not "Enough"—Feel Inadequate
• Positive Self-Image	• Negative Self-Image
• Reveal "Self" to Others	• Conceal "Self" from Others
Purposes	
• Approach to Issues is Freeing— working with others to understand issues and change them—solution focused vs. problem focused, strength exploration vs. Weakness	• Approach to Problem is "problem" emphasis; Controlling "fix it" orientation
• Focus on Larger Goals Search for authentic meaning; inner truth/purpose/vision	• Focus on Smaller Goals

BELIEFS THAT MAKE A DIFFERENCE

LEARNING ACTIVITY:
WALKING THE WALK: BELIEFS THAT MAKE A DIFFERENCE

Ends in View

This learning activity will provide you with opportunities to consider how your beliefs impact on your pedagogical practices.

Using the format set out by Combs in his study on teaching effectiveness, try to identify where your beliefs fit within these categories. Create a blank table using his headings, and fill it in using your knowledge about yourself in teaching/learning situations. Consider your readings, thoughts, and discussions about beliefs and values. Using the framework you developed based on Combs' work, identify areas where you need to reconsider your beliefs. Using this same framework, write goals for yourself for the remainder of the course. Your journal is a great place to consistently reflect on your progress.

Time Out for Reflection

Think about the following questions:

What is your reaction to Combs study?

Does it resonate with you?

What did you discover about your beliefs in relation to Combs' findings?

What is the orientation you bring to your own life problems? To others' problems?

BELIEFS AND ASSUMPTIONS ABOUT CARING SCIENCE CURRICULUM

The purpose of this section is to highlight the important role that beliefs, values, and assumptions play in guiding our thinking, behavior, and actions in general as we engage in the curriculum development process in general and, specifically, the influence they have on our pedagogical practices.

Beliefs and Assumptions About Humanity

Certain assumptions about humanity underlie a Caring Science curriculum. These assumptions acknowledge the following:

- People are unitary Beings and cannot be broken down into component parts. People experience the world as whole human beings and make meaning of the world as they experience it.
- People are able and evolving and everyone has their own learning journey. This assumption is based on the belief that people have the ability to identify their own needs, have inner wisdom to solve their own problems, and generally know what is best for them in a given situation. This assumption also recognizes that people are their own best resource and often need only support and/or understanding to better understand and respond to their health issue or problems.
- People are always situated. This assumption is closely related to the existential-phenomenological perspective that people are always situated in time and space and can best be understood within their own context. This refers to people's social, cultural, political, and historical background and experiences; it recognizes the impact of this context in relation to health choices.
- Individual and social responsibility for health and well-being is increasingly highlighted in local and global health discourse; acknowledging that expanded notions of health and well-being are distinct from the historic medical-technocure orientation to health as the absence of disease or illness.

Beliefs and Assumptions Related to Health and Healing

A Caring Science curriculum is based on the following assumptions about health and healing:

- Health is individually and subjectively defined and best understood by the person experiencing it. The person experiencing a health issue is in the best position to name it. Nurses cannot assume that all people experience health issues in the same way. Health and illness coexist and are not points on a continuum. People who are experiencing health issues or an illness often consider themselves healthy. This is particularly relevant for those people who experience chronic health challenges such as living with diabetes.

- There is a difference between curing and healing; curing seeks to eliminate disease, treat, remove, and diagnose. Curing is largely focusing on the body physical. Healing represents wholeness, oneness, unity of mindbodyspirit; healing is *"being-in-right-relation"* (Quinn, 1989); it honors and incorporates the human spirit, transcending the body/physical/material/medicine mindset.

- Diversity is valued and celebrated. Respect for differences is inherent in one's assumptions and beliefs, honoring differences of race, culture, sexual orientation, political orientation, or ways of thinking about or being-in-the-world.

- One of the greatest human needs is to be authentically heard and to authentically listen to another's story; thus, they are more able to hear and listen to their own inner wisdom, to detect their own best solutions for health and healing.

From these broader philosophical, scientific, and spiritual perspectives, one realizes that someone may be cured of a disease but not be healed. Healing, in contrast to curing, is based upon the internal meaning, the inner subjective experiences, and held by the individual person and all the processes and thoughts held in relation to the disease, the treatment, and outcomes. Healing is an inner process, whereas curing is an outer treatment process. With this level of awareness, someone may, in the process of dying, experience the ultimate healing. That is, if they are helped to die peacefully, having taken care of "unfinished business" and *"being in right relation"* with self and other, their dying is a peaceful and sacred transition. Perhaps, it is the ultimate healing.

A Caring Science Curriculum Reflects a Teacher's Belief in

- power and primacy of people in-relation, power of human consciousness, human imagination, and human spirit;
- the inner resources, the individual interests, and passionate scholarly questions and wonderings as key components in teaching-learning and in health-illness processes and outcomes;

- all student questions are considered sacred, no question is treated as trivial, as any and all questions reflect the inner learning processes of the student;
- wholeness, harmony and beauty; connectedness/oneness of all; Beauty inner Truth;
- the unitary wholeness of human and environment and the larger universe;
- ways of knowing and teaching-learning that incorporate not only rational, cognitive, and technical empirics but also call upon aesthetic values, moral ideals, intuition, personal knowing, joy of process discovery, passion, and spiritual-metaphysical dimensions;
- the context of inter-subjectivity, inter-human events, processes, relationships; and human-environment energetic patterns within universal field;
- an ontology of evolving consciousness, human freedom, release of human spirit—while adhering to caring as a moral ideal and absolute value for sustaining human dignity; and authentic relationships in education and practice; and
- a worldview for human-evolutionary destiny that is open (Watson, 1989, p. 52)

In summary, these basic, identified beliefs and assumptions underlie a Caring Science curriculum. Making explicit such basic assumptions provides the disciplinary foundation for education and professional practice, as well as for scholarly inquiry. This explicit disciplinary Caring Science orientation to education and teaching-learning seeks to release and tap into inner resources, the human spirit; in order to inspire, invite, empower, and emancipate student and educator, as well as patients. Finally, Caring Science seeks to preserve human dignity and honor the whole person for learning *and* healing; it is open to inner exploration for meaning and personal knowing, and, thus, the transformation and evolution of human consciousness.
As noted by Clark: (Clark, 2010, p. 50):

> As we heal our individual selves, [our classrooms], small workplaces, communities, and our larger systems, we can partake of the Great Awakening universal change process in the nursing profession . . . realize our interconnectedness and take our profession into a place of sacred autonomous practices . . .

EMANCIPATORY KNOWING:
STUDENT–TEACHER DYNAMICS

The next section uncovers how deeply held beliefs and assumptions play out in student-teacher–student dynamics, in turn affecting classroom relations, emancipatory learning, and knowing.

> It is vital to de-professionalize the public debate on matters that vitally affect the lives of ordinary people.
>
> (Arundhati Roy, Indian writer-activist, 2001)

Chinn and Kramer, in their classic work on theory and knowledge development (2008, 7th ed.), point out that through *emancipatory knowing* (our emphasis) nurses gain the ability to critique and analyze barriers of unfair and unjust conditions, and the complexity of social and political contexts, thus becoming agents of change to improve human life.

A Caring Science curriculum holds underlying beliefs and assumptions about power-control dynamics. The core assumption is based on the notion that there is reciprocity between power, knowledge, and control, and that, in order for there to be more equitable relationships, there is shared power. Thus, everyone benefits as they share their knowledge and in turn hold authentic power with others. Authentic power is shared power; it is power with, not power over. It does not negate faculty or nurses' responsibilities, skills, or knowledge. It also means standing in one's own power, one's own truth and integrity, without succumbing to other's power position, authoritarian control, and so on.

We still acknowledge the reality that there is a difference between having authority and being authoritarian; the teacher has authority by the nature of his/her position; however, that position does not justify an authoritarian, power-control stance toward knowledge, toward students and toward control of knowledge. In a Caring Science curriculum, students also have authority in their own knowing and experiences that can be shared and jointly critiqued for deeper knowledge. As Canales and others emphasize, "emancipatory learning helps to situate ourselves in the center of another's experience, while recognizing and respecting our differences" (in Canales, 2010, p. 31; Aptheker, 1989, p. 60)—not as separate, but as a reflection of the diversity of our shared human condition.

Issues of differences and power can be thought through and further critiqued within a Caring Science curriculum. As Mohanty (2003) points out, there is a need to think relationally (e.g., Caring Science is about honoring each individual as a unique person, embracing a relational ethical-ontological worldview and starting point) about questions of power, equality, justice, and the need to be inclusive. We know from our shared life experiences, as well as from the wisdom traditions across time, that we are all connected through our shared humanity and our sharing the Planet Earth and its precious resources.

Once again it is helpful to remind ourselves that everyone is situated in a given personal, relational, historical, cultural, deep phenomenal life-experience context. This backdrop needs to be considered, as each context of self and other is deeply rooted in a personal inner life contextual phenomenal field of history and meaning. In a Caring Science framework, the basic tenet is that one person's level of humanity reflects on the other and at the deeply human level, we are all one and connected through our shared humanity (Watson, 2002, 2006, 2008a). As the poet Maya Angelou reminds us in a major address, "I am a Human Being and nothing Human is alien to me" (in Watson, 2008b, p. 55)—thus if one person is put down, so am I; "likewise if the other person's human spirit is lifted up, so is mine" (Watson, 2008b, p. 56).

Within a Caring Science curriculum, it is important to uncover more pervasive issues of power/control/knowledge/social justice. What is of deeper concern regarding power relations in education and clinical care practices are the more fundamental issues of knowledge/epistemology as power and, thus, epistemology as ethic (Palmer, 2004).

EPISTEMOLOGY AS ETHIC: ANOTHER TURN IN POWER RELATIONS IN EDUCATION AND PEDAGOGY*

Within a critique of knowledge and education, curriculum and learning, we have a new awareness, an awakening to the fact that every epistemology (ways of knowing and what counts as knowledge) becomes an ethic (Palmer, 2004). A fundamental conflict has prevailed within our institutions of higher learning that has already caught up with us in the Western world of science and professionalism. Everything has consequences. The types and ways of teaching and learning that have prevailed at the cognitive, intellectual, rational level alone are formative to our human development; they are shaping the lives of human beings and forming, informing, or deforming our mind-sets and actions as people and as professionals. As Palmer (2004, p. 2) profoundly

---

*Excerpt reprinted from Watson, 2008a, chapter 20.

asked, "What ethical formation and deformation has this approach to education created in our lives?" suggesting overtly a relationship between our knowledge and violence: the violence of knowledge (and language of power, control, domination, superiority). This form of knowledge development as often practiced in institutions of higher learning has "lent itself to subtle and pervasive forms of violence," to our personal, social, and professional ontological being, our epistemology informing our ethics, our human mode of living (2004, p. 2).

By "violence," Palmer means more subtle forms than dropping a bomb or hitting someone physically. Rather, he refers to violence associated with "violating the integrity" of the other, whether the other is the earth, another human being, or another culture. This mode of learning and knowledge is tied up with the Western academy emphasis on three dominant ways of thinking, teaching, and learning, which according to Palmer (2004) are intended to guide our professional and personal lives: "objective, analytic, and experimental."

Each of these three dominant ways of learning, of valuing, of teaching, of knowing is critiqued by Palmer in his classic paper presented at the 2004 U.S. Fetzer Institute–sponsored conference, "21st Century Learning Initiatives." He points out the misguided myth that one cannot know anything truly well unless it is held at arm's length, at a distance, at great remove from self—thus perpetuating a chasm between the knower and the known. This myth reinforces the belief that knowledge is tainted, distorted, and untrustworthy if close to the individual; thus, one cannot possibly generate valid knowledge from a personal connection with the data or information.

Objectivism as Mythic Epistemology—Epistemology-as-Ethic

Within this mythic epistemological system of knowledge, of learning, of valuing, of teaching as objective, Palmer reminds us that we create a profound fear of subjectivity, a fear of relatedness, of entering into a relationship with that which we know. Using the metaphors of war, he points out different explanations of the approaches related to objectivity and subjectivity. For example, we can try to detach ourselves from what is happening in an objective medical diagnosis, making disease a war of conquest to fight against the body, the disease. Further, it is safer to detach and separate self from other experiencing person. However, the subjective experience cannot be held at emotional–spiritual arm's length from the medical impersonal analysis; our world may be turned upside down, but the medical–clinical gaze is on the disease, the fight to win the war through correct diagnosis and treatment with cure the ultimate end, often at all costs. We all eventually, come face to face with subjective evidence of our vulnerability and connectedness with our inner life world, our very humanity.

With the thin line of separation and connectedness between objective and subjective clinical professional relationships, one can begin to see how our limited view of how we think about objective knowledge crosses over into ethics.

We cannot therefore justify "turning our face away" from self or others who are different from us or distant from us.

Objectivity for its own sake and the mythology of rightness from a clinical (distanced) point of view can create cruelty if we are not able to accurately acknowledge and portray how events, knowledge, and experiences really exist/coexist in our world.

For its part, the objectivist mythology, whether in medical science per se or in terms of clinical war metaphors used for personal life events, is a distortion both of reality and knowledge—certainly a distortion of values and a distortion of science and how science is done. Palmer (2004) helps us remember: great knowing and great learning are not simply done objectively. Paradoxically, great knowing and learning constitute a dance between the objective and subjective, between intimacy and distance, between the personal, inner life world and the outer, professional-political domain. This is true in all disciplines, not just nursing. The mythology of objectivism is "more about [power] and control over the world, or over each other [or a given phenomenon], more a mythology of power than a real epistemology that reflects how real knowing proceeds" (p. 4). As such, perpetuating this mythology of objectivism does not help us to see that "every epistemology becomes an ethic" (Palmer, p. 2) and affects how we value and see the different phenomena in our world.

Nightingale as Exemplar of Understanding "Epistemology as Ethic"

The story of Nightingale and her hands-on approach to knowing is a historic as well as a modern example of the "dance" of great knowing, the paradoxical integration of the subjective and objective. She skillfully wove together objective data and subjective visions, a personal sense of calling for her mission and outer-world life's work that transcended any objectivist logic of her era. Yet her internal ethics guided her approach to knowing, to valuing, to teaching, and to learning. She is arguably an exemplar of living the paradox of oneness with her being, knowing, doing in the world. This is not to say that we must agree with everything she said and did, but it is worth remembering that her underlying beliefs, assumptions, and weltanschauung (worldview) was largely what motivated her actions as one of the founders of modern nursing.

The Analytic and Experimental as Mythic Epistemology

Just as objectivism is a mythology yet can destructively become our ethic, ethos, and mind-set for teaching, learning, scholarship, and so on, Parker Palmer (2004) pointed out the same misstep with the notion that "analytic" and "experimental" mean "being scientific." Analytic, as he makes explicit, means that once you have objectified a phenomenon as something to be studied, you are then free to cut it into little pieces to see how it works; to break it down into parts, hold it at a distance, analyze it, and thus understand it. Palmer used this cutting-things-up phenomenon in order to look at, to understand, something "objectively," as a metaphor for what education often does to the human mind and human heart and human soul—the human experience in its totality. This cutting up approach is the same as trying to describe and appreciate a rose, by cutting it up into little pieces. The same is true about humans and any human phenomena. The pieces never can depict and capture understanding, beauty, appreciation, majesty, or even knowledge of the whole "rose."

Palmer argues that this great facility for taking things apart, dissecting them to the point that one cannot know the original, is a form of violence in that it cultivates a lack of sensitivity and little capacity for putting things back together, including the human heart.

The same is true for the myth of "experimental," in that the mythology of objectivity, analytic, sets up mythological imprints that suggest that once things are objectified, dissected into parts, we are free to experiment. This focus in turn leads us to justify reducing a human to the moral status of object so we can objectively know, study, experiment, and conduct science.

This form of experimentation with humans and nature leads us to seek designs with what we think the world should be like, to control and dominate the outcome, so to speak, with our logic, our distant data, and our moving things around from their original form. We do this without paying attention to potentially destructive outcomes for self, society, humanity, the environment, and nature alike.

In summary, this section has introduced beliefs and assumptions as the starting point that underpins curriculum, approaches to humanity, to relations, to knowledge, power, and emancipatory education. We made more explicit what is meant by Caring Science, its assumptions, beliefs, and nature of the politics, policies, and dynamics that affect and can alter educational practices. Conventional myths identified by Parker Palmer (2004), world-renowned educator, helped us reveal how set beliefs both subtly, and overtly, permeate our approaches toward self and other, toward teaching-learning, toward education, and curriculum. This Caring Science critique shifts the discourse from conventional minds and mindsets of education, of nursing, of caring, of teaching to learning, to emancipatory approaches, to knowledge and all ways of knowing. This shift offers a new turn in nursing education; and ultimately invites the human spirit, the head-heart, soul, and love of nursing, a love of humanity, back into nursing, back into our educational programs, and back into our world.

Time Out for Reflection

How does Caring Science epistemology differ from conventional views of knowledge?

How can epistemology be/become an ethic?

What are the prevailing myths of knowledge, knowing, and epistemology?

How would you describe issues of power-control operating in your personal life world?

Now reflect on your experiences of power-control as a student, as a teacher, and as a nurse.

REFERENCES

Aptheker, B. (1989). *Tapestries of life: Women's work, women's consciousness and the meaning of daily life.* Amherst, MA: The University of Massachusetts Press.

Canales, M. (2010). Othering: Difference understood? *Advances in Nursing Science, 33*(1), 15–34.

Chinn, P. L., & Kramer, M. K. (2008). *Integrated theory and knowledge development in nursing* (7th ed.). St. Louis, MO: Mosby.

Clark, C. S. (2010). The nursing shortage as a community transformational opportunity. *Advances in Nursing Science, 33*(1), 35–52.

Combs, A. (1971). *Helping relationships: Basic concepts for the helping professions.* Boston: Allyn & Bacon.

Combs, A. (1979). *Myths in education.* Boston: Allyn & Bacon.

Combs, A. (1982). *Personal approach to teaching: Beliefs that make a difference.* Boston: Allyn & Bacon.

Egan, G. (1985). *The skilled helper.* Monterey, CA: Brooks-Cole.

Mohanty, C. T. (2003). *Feminism without borders: Decolonizing theory: Practicing solidarity.* Durham, NC: Duke University Press.

Palmer, P. (2004). *The violence of our knowledge: Toward a spirituality of higher education. 21st learning initiative.* Kalamazoo, MI: Fetzer Institute.

Quinn, J. F. (1989). On healing, wholeness and the Haelan effect. *Nursing and Health Care, 10*(10), 553–556.

Roy, A. (2001). *Power politics.* Cambridge, MA: South End Press.

Watson, J. (1989). A new paradigm of curriculum development. In E. O. Bevis & J. Watson (Eds.), *Toward a caring curriculum.* New York: NLN.

Watson, J. (2002). Intentionality and caring-healing consciousness: A practice of transpersonal nursing. *Holistic Nursing Practice, 16*(4), 12–19.

Watson, J. (2006). *Caring science as sacred science.* Philadelphia: FA Davis.

Watson, J. (2008a). *Nursing: The philosophy and science of caring.* (New Rev. ed.). Boulder, CO: University Press of Colorado.

Watson, J. (2008b). Social justice and human caring: A model of caring science as a hopeful paradigm for moral justice for humanity. *Creative Nursing, 14*(2), 54–61.

II
AN EMANCIPATORY RELATIONAL PEDAGOGY FOR CARING SCIENCE CURRICULA

*If the (teacher) is indeed wise he does not bid you enter the house
of his wisdom, but rather leads you to the threshold of your own mind.*
—*The Prophet, Khalil Gibran*

I N THIS UNIT, WE PRESENT our emancipatory relational pedagogical framework for a Caring Science curriculum. This framework integrates four essential elements that when taken together create a dynamic relational inquiry process. These elements are described separately, but in reality they work synergistically to support the theory and philosophy of Caring Science.

Chapter 3 introduces the concept of pedagogy, identifies our conceptualization of pedagogy, and provides a rationale for why this type of pedagogy is required for a Caring Science curriculum. It describes our emancipatory pedagogy as relational inquiry, provides an overview of our emancipatory relational pedagogy including a description of the four essential components of this pedagogical framework. Also, this introductory chapter describes our conceptualization of knowledge and knowledge development as used in this pedagogy.

Each subsequent chapter in this unit provides a detailed description of each of the essential components that comprise this pedagogy and gives examples of how to develop this component as part of an emancipatory relational pedagogy. The intention is that students can examine and critique this framework and develop their own emancipatory relational framework for a Caring Science curriculum.

Chapter 4 provides an overview of element one, creating caring collaborative relationships. Chapter 5 introduces the second element, engaging in critical caring dialogue, Chapter 6 describes the third element, reflection-in-action, and Chapter 7 describes the final component, creating a culture of caring.

3

Emancipatory Pedagogy: The Transformation of Consciousness Through Relational Inquiry

The academy is not paradise. But learning is a place where
paradise can be created. The classroom, with all its limitations,
remains a location of possibility. In that field of possibility we have
the opportunity to labor for freedom, to demand of our selves and
our comrades an openness of mind and heart that allows us to face
reality even as we begin to move beyond boundaries, to transgress.
—hooks, 1994, p. 207

I N THIS INITIAL CHAPTER OF THE UNIT, we begin by setting the context for our pedagogical framework. We describe some of the historical educational theories that have influenced the development of our current pedagogy. We continue by examining some definitions of pedagogy that are commonly used, and we describe our conception of it. Further, we explain why we claim our emancipatory pedagogy to be relational inquiry, and we describe our views of knowledge, various forms of inquiry, and knowledge development, all of which are inherent in our pedagogy. We end the chapter by introducing our emancipatory relational pedagogy and its essential components.

EDUCATIONAL THEORETICAL PERSPECTIVES: INFLUENCES ON THE DEVELOPMENT OF OUR EMANCIPATORY PEDAGOGY

Caring science curricula can be considered in many ways; they are **not** dependent on a single theoretical perspective or view. There are many educational perspectives and nursing educational theories that are

47

congruent with a Caring Science curriculum and we encourage you to explore them. Several of these educational views have influenced our current thinking about our emancipatory relational pedagogy. The four described below are important to us because they are concurrent with a Caring Science curricula development process and its related pedagogies.

A Perceptual View

Combs (1982) describes learning as a deeply personal experience that is always concerned with the discovery of personal meaning. His theory of teaching/learning is based on perceptual psychology. The theory postulates that an individual's behavior is understood to be the direct consequence of the total field of personal meanings existing at that instant. "These meanings extend far beyond sensory experience to include such perceptions as: beliefs, values, feelings, hopes, desires, and the personal ways in which people regard themselves and others" (p. 30).

Combs suggests that effective learning always consists of two aspects: the acquisition of new information or experience, and the individual's personal discovery of the meaning of the experience. He, therefore, sees teaching/learning as having three components:

- *Creating a safe environment for learning.* From Combs' perspective, the teacher is responsible to create a learning environment that is free from threat and yet is challenging. He contends that, because learning is a deeply personal experience and thus requires self-exploration, people must put themselves in what they might perceive to be vulnerable positions in order to have significant learning experiences. The teacher must create an atmosphere that encourages daring and venturing forth. "What ever narrows or hampers the exploration of ideas and the discovery of self must be rigorously eliminated from the teacher-education process" (1982, p. 34).

- *Providing new information or experiences.* Most teachers concentrate considerable effort and energy on this aspect of teaching. Combs suggests that **the way** in which information or experience is delivered is of utmost importance. He contends that it is often assumed that learning is a simple process of presentation and absorption. "The genius of good teaching lies in the capacity to fire the imagination" (1982, p. 51). Teachers need to feel passionate about their subject matter and their students.

- *Facilitating the discovery of personal meaning.* Combs believes that this aspect of teaching is often overlooked, yet it is the most critical. He suggests that learning is deeply personal and that, for information to be translated to knowledge, learners must be engaged in a process of discovering the meaning of information or experience for them personally. He states that "any information will affect a person's behavior only to the extent that s/he has it's meaning for him" (1982, p. 62). So, facilitating the discovery of personal meaning involves encouraging learners to struggle with ideas, share their thinking, make mistakes, experiment with new ideas and skills, and actively participate in all aspects of learning.

Combs cautions that teachers are often very good at the first two components but tend to ignore the final and most significant component—the discovery of personal meaning.

Combs asserts that it not the skills, knowledge, or methods of teachers that make them effective but rather the beliefs that they hold.

A Humanistic View

Rogers' views (1969) are closely related to those of Combs. However, Rogers, a humanistic psychologist, has a strong opinion about the role of teaching, contending that the teaching aspect of the educational process is "vastly unimportant and overrated." He suggests that to focus on teaching leads us to consider the wrong issues and ask the wrong questions.

> As soon as we focus on teaching, the question arises, what shall we teach? What, from our superior vantage point, does the other need to know? . . . What should the course cover? . . . This notion of coverage is based on the assumption that what is taught is what is learned. . . . One does not need research to provide evidence that this is false. One needs only to talk to a few students. (p. 104)

Rogers contends that you cannot **teach** anyone anything and that we should place our emphasis in education on the facilitation of **learning**. In describing this possibility, he states:

> When I have been able to transform a group—and here I mean all the members of the group, myself included—into a

community of learners, then the excitement has been almost beyond belief. To free curiosity; to permit individuals to go charging off in a new direction dictated by their own interest; to unleash the sense of inquiry; to open everything to questioning and exploration; to recognize that everything is in a process of change—here is the experience I can never forget. (p. 105)

Rogers contends that significant learning does not rely upon teaching skills, scholarly knowledge, curriculum planning, or a particular theoretical perspective. Rather, it is dependent upon certain attitudinal qualities that exist in the personal relationship between the facilitator and learners. Rogers identifies three qualities that facilitate learning:

- *Realness in the facilitator of learning.* This means that the *humanness,* the *personhood,* of the facilitator is present in the relationship with learners. The facilitator is aware of who she/he is and what she/he feels and relates person-to-person in interactions with learners. "There is no sterile facade. Here is a vital person, with convictions, with feelings . . . a transparent realness . . . that makes her an exciting facilitator of learning". (p. 107)

- *Prizing, acceptance, and trust.* This attitude involves a nonpossessive caring about the learner and the acceptance of each individual as worthy and valuable in his/her own right. This attitude permits the facilitator to accept learners' occasional apathy, anger, or disappointment in a learning situation. "What we are describing is a prizing of the learner as an imperfect human being with many feelings, many potentialities" (p. 109). It is an essential trust in the capacity of humankind.

- *Empathic understanding.* "Being empathic is a complex, demanding and strong—yet subtle and gentle—way of being" (p. 142). Empathic understanding has several facets, including a deep, committed way of listening that momentarily suspends our prejudices so that we can truly hear the other's experiences; momentarily entering the perceptual world of the other; sensing what is present without it being spoken; and communicating our understanding in ways that honor the other's experience. "When the teacher has the ability to understand the student's reactions from the inside, has a sensitive awareness of the way the process of education and learning seems to the student, then again the likelihood of significant learning is increased" (p. 111).

An Emancipatory View

Freire (1972) focuses on education and pedagogy in his discussions of teaching and learning. He describes a pedagogy for liberation by contrasting it to a traditional *banking* approach to education. Freire confirms the notions espoused by Combs, Rogers, and others by suggesting that, for education to be truly liberating, the student–teacher contradiction must be resolved. The resolution of this contradiction requires a transformation of the typical dichotomy of teacher as dominant and student as subservient to a partnership that recognizes that both parties are teachers and learners simultaneously.

Freire further suggests that education must focus on problem posing rather than on problem solving if we are to successfully engage students in a process of learning-to-learn rather than one of accumulating information. In other words, we must engage in emancipatory education rather than in a transfer-of-knowledge pedagogy. "Liberating education consists of acts of cognition, not transferals of information" (Freire, 1972, p. 53).

The notion of power is a critical aspect of Freire's pedagogy. As he explains, "If teachers or students exercised the power to remake knowledge in the classroom, then they would be asserting their power to remake society" (p. 10). According to Freire, ". . . the lecture-based, passive curriculum is not simply poor pedagogical practice. It is the teaching model most compatible with promoting the dominant authority in society and with disempowering students" (p. 10). Therefore, the touchstone of Freire's pedagogy for liberation is raising critical consciousness in order to transform society. Besides being an act of knowing, education is also a political act.

> That is why no pedagogy is neutral. They all have a form and a
> content that relate to power in society, that construct one kind
> of society or another, and they all have society relationships
> in the classroom that confirm or challenge domination. (p. 13)

A Nursing View

Bevis and Watson (1989) developed a transformative caring pedagogy for nursing education. Their emancipatory approach calls for encouragement of self-reflection wherein the educators can come in touch with their own humanity and encourage the release of the human spirit in teaching-learning-caring processes that must be considered in nursing education. Through this process, nurse educators seek to facilitate learning associated with human health and healing processes and expert human caring practices.

Bevis and Watson redefine curriculum to be "those transactions and interactions that take place between teachers and students and among students, with the intent that learning take place" (p. 72). Although they describe education as an elusive concept, they call for an approach to education that "appeals to freeing the human potential, an approach that allows one to develop not only rational and moral capacities, but emotional, expressive, intuitive, aesthetic, personal capacities and to bring about one's full self to bear with one's life work—in this instance, the work of human caring" (p. 47). They further suggest that the teacher's main purpose is to provide the climate, the structure, and the dialogue that promotes praxis (Bevis & Watson, 1989; Watson, 2000).

Bevis and Watson suggest that education should have as its goal graduating students who are independent, self-directed, self moti-vated, and lifelong learners, with questioning minds and a familiarity with inquiring approaches to learning.

These four theoretical educational perspectives have influenced our thinking about pedagogy and the development of our emancipatory relational pedagogy. Although we fully endorse these perspectives, it is our intention to expand and synthesize these conceptualizations of education to more fully embrace the most recent developments and understandings of pedagogies that are situated in a nursing caring sci-ence paradigm.

PEDAGOGY: WHAT IS IT?

The term pedagogy is given various definitions and interpretations. Webster's Dictionary defines pedagogy as the art and science of teach-ing (Webster). Chinn (1989) describes pedagogy as "the actions we take in the learning environment, the materials we use, how we use them, and the attitudes we convey" (p. 9); whereas Gore (1993) proposes that pedagogy is the means by which knowledge is produced and trans-mitted by practical instructional approaches (practices) in addition to the articulation of a social vision underlying the approach to educa-tion. Although the term pedagogy is often used synonymously with the process of teaching/learning, Ironside (2001) argues that pedagogy is more than teaching because it involves a way of thinking about and the comportment within education. Kenway and Modra (1992) also postulate that, when it is used in its broadest sense, pedagogy, often associated with the teaching of children, includes what is taught, how it is learned, and the nature of knowledge and learning itself, including "what counts as knowledge, how knowledge is produced, negotiated, transformed and realized in the interaction/relations between the teacher, the learner and the knowledge itself" (p. 140).

Why Does a Caring Science Curriculum Require a Relational Pedagogy?

Our current view is that pedagogy, especially an emancipatory pedagogy, is a relational inquiry process (explained in further detail below) that facilitates the transformation of consciousness (see Figures 3.1 and 3.2) through which learning and deeper insight occurs. Transformation of consciousness within this context helps us realize that, ultimately, all knowledge becomes personal knowledge—it is the discovery of the personal meaning of knowledge. This occurs when knowledge is incorporated and integrated, with deep understanding and inner subjective knowing that connects with personal meaning. This process of insight and integration with a deeper connection of meaning for "personally knowing," results in transformation of consciousness.

While the earlier definitions of pedagogy, especially the latter two, capture much of what we believe to be relevant to a Caring Science, emancipatory pedagogy as a relational inquiry process, we believe that some critical aspects are overlooked. From our broader perspective, important relationships and interactions reveal themselves.

It is our view that learning occurs at the juncture or intersection when the teacher and students are in a caring relationship and are cocreating knowledge. They are engaged in a process of transformational learning in which they cocreate knowledge through the complex caring relational process: relation with subject matter; relation with own ideas and personal meaning; through relation with peers/classmates/social-political dynamics; and through caring student–teacher relationship among other relational dynamics of inner subjective experiences. Therefore, we believe that learning occurs in the intersection of the complexity of caring relationships that lead to new insights, new knowledge, and deeper understandings, resulting in the transformation of consciousness. Transformation of consciousness includes an evolution of consciousness, in that both student and teacher experience a higher dimension of integration from before, including a higher consciousness and repatterning of old into something new.

From our caring relational perspective, one aspect of the pedagogical process is not valued over another, and the teacher and student are engaged in a mutual inquiry process of learning—a relational inquiry process. In contrast to more traditional *banking* conceptualizations of teaching and learning in which the teacher is seen as the transmitter of information, this perspective does not permit the teacher to be viewed as an expert (see Figure 3.1) with knowledge to impart, the student to be a passive receipt of the knowledge, or the knowledge itself to be seen as merely information to be transmitted. This conceptualization of pedagogy highlights the complexity of the relational nature of the teaching/learning process and the teacher/learner relationship. Therefore, this perspective shows that emancipatory pedagogy is relational inquiry.

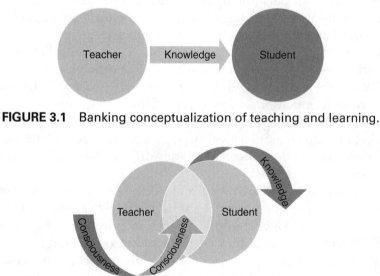

FIGURE 3.1   Banking conceptualization of teaching and learning.

FIGURE 3.2   Emancipatory pedagogy as a relational inquiry process.
Source: Adapted from Hills, M. (2000). *A Workshop Report:* Brazilian Congress on Collective Health, Salvador, Brazil.

Why Does a Caring Science Curriculum Require an Emancipatory Pedagogy?

As we nursing educators begin to embrace Caring Science as a philosophical and theoretical foundation upon which to teach nursing, we must embrace a pedagogy that is congruent with this orientation. We argue that, in order to support Caring Science as the foundation of nursing, nurse educators need to develop pedagogical approaches that liberate, emancipate, and empower future nurses. As Bevis (2000) explains:

> . . . without emancipation, education is an oppressive tool. It is an assembly line industry producing nurse-workers who on average follow the status quo. They may make waves, but they stay within the rules while living lives that are circumscribed by the inflexibility of large medical empire-bureaucracies and bear the inevitable stamp of banality and mediocrity. Emancipatory education encourages learners to ask the unaskable, confront injustices and oppression and be active agents in their lives and in their work (p. 162).

Combining a relational perspective with an emancipatory one aligns the teacher and the student and together they engage with the information to be learned. As Freire explains, "through dialogue the teacher-of-the-students and the students-of-the-teacher cease to exist and a new term emerges teacher/student-with-student/teachers. The teacher is no longer merely the one who teaches, but one whom is himself taught in dialogue with the students, who in their turn, while being taught, also teach. They become jointly responsible for a process in which all grow. . . . Here no one teaches another, nor is one self taught" (p. 53).

So, if we want to graduate nurses who embrace caring as their moral compass that guides all their actions and who are independent thinkers with confidence in their ability to make clinical judgments, we must educate them within a truly *emancipatory relational* pedagogy. We believe deeply and passionately that people are able, and that our responsibility as teachers is to create ambiguity, to challenge taken-for-granted assumptions, and to create an environment in which learners feel free to wrestle with ideas, challenge us and other learners, share half-baked ideas, and engage in critical dialogue about the issues at hand. An emancipatory relational pedagogy accomplishes this goal.

KNOWLEDGE: FROM AN EMANCIPATORY RELATIONAL PEDAGOGICAL PERSPECTIVE

Before describing our emancipatory relational pedagogy, we think it is important to mention our views on knowledge. There is so much that could be said about knowledge development and ways of knowing (Carper, 1978; Belinky, Clinchy, Goldenberger, & Tarule, 1986) but, as these concepts are well developed elsewhere, we will confine our comments to aspects of knowledge that are directly related to an emancipatory relational pedagogy.

Paradigm, Ontology, Epistemology, and Axiology

Our emancipatory relation pedagogy is based on a participatory paradigm (Heron & Reason, 1997) that includes a subjective-objective ontology; an extended epistemology and an axiology that values practical knowing and human flourishing. The meaning and importance of these terms in relation to knowledge development is described in this section of the chapter.

Participatory Paradigm

A paradigm is "a set of basic beliefs (or metaphysics) that deals with ultimates or first principles. It represents a worldview that defines, for its holder, the nature of the world, the individual's place in it, and the range of possible relationships to that world and its parts, as, for example, cosmologies and theologies do" (Guba & Lincoln, 1994, p. 105). A Caring Science curriculum and an emancipatory relational pedagogy is based in participatory paradigm that rests on the belief that reality is interplay between the given cosmos and the mind. The mind "creatively participates with [the cosmos] and can only know it in terms of its constructs, whether affective, imaginable, conceptual or practical" . . . (Heron & Reason, 1997, p. 10) "Mind and the given cosmos are engaged in a creative dance, so that what emerges as reality is the fruit of an interaction of the given cosmos and the way the mind engages with it" (Heron & Reason, 1997, p. 279). As Skolimowski (1994) states; "we always partake of what we describe so our reality is a product of the dance between our individual and collective mind and 'what is there', the amorphous primordial giveness of the universe" (p. 20). This participative worldview is at the heart of the emancipatory relational pedagogy that emphasizes participation as a core strategy.

Subjective–Objective Ontology

Ontology refers to the form and nature of reality and what can be known about it (Guba & Lincoln, 1994). In contrast to more orthodox pedagogies that are based on an objective ontology and that utilize traditional teaching methods to impart knowledge, an emancipatory relational pedagogy endorses a subjective-objective ontology.

A subjective-objective ontology means that there is "underneath our literate abstraction, a deeply participatory relation to things, people and to the earth, a felt reciprocity" (Abram, 1996, p. 124). As Heron and Reason (1997) explain, this encounter is transactional and interactive. "To touch, see, or hear something or someone does not tell us either about our self all on its own or about a being out there all on its own. It tells us about a being in a state of interrelation and co-presence with us. Our subjectivity feels the participation of what is there and is illuminated by it", . . . (p. 279). So an emancipatory relational pedagogy is interested in the cocreation of knowledge as we together investigate our understandings and meanings as we experience them in the world.

Extended Epistemology

Epistemology, the branch of philosophy that studies the nature of knowledge, deals with the nature of the relationship between the knower and what can be known. Often, the word knowledge conjures up a notion of factual information, facts, and theories that exist to explain phenomena. An emancipatory relational pedagogy embraces an extended epistemology that includes at least four types of knowledge and that endorses the primacy of practical knowing. Teachers and students participate in the "known" and generate knowledge in at least four interdependent ways—experiential, presentational, propositional, and practical (Heron & Reason, 1997).

Experiential Knowing

Experiential knowing refers to direct encounters with persons, places, or things. "It is knowing through participatory, empathic resonance with a being, so that as the knower, I feel both attuned with it and distinct from it" (Reason, 1997, p. 281). Experiential knowing incorporates the participatory nature of perception as postulated by Husserl (1964) and Merleau-Ponty (1962). "Hardness and softness, roughness and smoothness, moonlight and sunlight, present themselves to us not as sensory contents but as certain kinds of symbiosis, certain ways the outside has of invading us and certain ways we have of meeting the invasion" (Merleau-Ponty, 1962, p. 317). Experiential knowing is "lived experience of the mutual co-determination of person and world" (Heron, 1997, p. 164).

Presentational Knowing

Presentational knowing is grounded in experiential knowing and is the way we represent our experiences through spatio-temporal images such as drawing, writing, dance, art, or stories. "These forms symbolize both our felt attunement with the world and the primary meaning embedded in our enactment of its appearing" (Polkinghorne, 1988; Reason, 1988, p. 281).

Empirical Knowing

Empirical knowing is factual knowledge: knowing about something conceptually. This type of knowledge is usually expressed in terms of statements, facts, or theories. This way of knowing is of utmost importance in more orthodox pedagogies. In an emancipatory relational pedagogy, propositional knowing is seen as interdependent with the other three ways of knowing.

Practical Knowing

Practical knowing has primacy in an emancipatory relational pedagogy. Practical knowing is knowing how to do something—it is knowledge in action. "Practical knowledge, knowing how, is the consummation, the fulfillment, of the knowledge quest" (Heron, 1997, p. 34). This form of knowing synthesizes our conceptualizations and experiences into action (practice). It becomes a part of our being in the world.

Each form of knowing is, to some degree, autonomous and can be understood and can function on its own. However, of interest in this book is the interdependent nature of these four ways of knowing. Practical knowing, knowledge-in-action, is grounded in propositional, presentational, and experiential knowing (Heron, 1997). Intentional action or change is practical knowing. Consequently, change can be thought of as being based on evidence from all four ways of knowing. In emancipatory relational pedagogy, as nursing teachers and learners acquire knowledge through action and reflection, they build theory (propositional knowing) from practice about what constitutes *good* nursing practice. Teachers and students test these theories in the real world of their practice and reflect on their experiences in relation to propositional knowing. The more congruent their four ways of knowing are, the more valid the evidence for nursing practice.

Before turning to a discussion of axiology, it is pertinent to further consider this relationship of theory to practice as it is critical to the development of knowledge development from an emancipatory relational pedagogical perspective. We refer to this relationship as *praxis*.

PRAXIS—THE RELATIONSHIP OF THEORY TO PRACTICE IN KNOWLEDGE DEVELOPMENT

Theory is often talked about as if it belongs in the world of the academy; some form of abstraction that is separate from our day-to-day lives. But, simply put, theory is an explanation of phenomena, and it is our contention that theory is implicit in **all** human action and is critical in developing knowledge for nursing practice. "Only theory can give us access to the unexpected questions and ways of changing situations from within" (Schratz & Walker, 1995, p. 107). The relationship of theory to practice is key in an emancipatory relational pedagogy. As Lewin (1947) declared many years ago, "there is nothing so practical as a good theory and the best place to find a good theory is by investigating interesting problems in everyday life" (p. 149) (or nursing practice).

In contrast to more orthodox pedagogies, an emancipatory relational pedagogy does not see theory as something that is known and that "informs" practice. As van Manen (1990) suggests "practice (or life) comes first and theory comes later as a result of reflection" (p. 15). In an emancipatory relational pedagogy, it is the cycling through the iterations of action and reflection, in which experiential knowing and propositional knowing are considered in relation to practical knowing that creates praxis and that generates new knowledge for future practice. This process grounds practice in theory rather than applying theory to practice. So often, in nursing education, we teach nursing theory and then provide practice experience and encourage students to apply what they have learned in the classroom to the clinical practice setting. An emancipatory relational pedagogy recognizes the reflective nature of this learning process by drawing theory from practice, reflecting on it, and taking it back to practice.

This notion of praxis is a fundamental concept in Freire's work and is fundamental to an emancipatory relational pedagogy. Praxis does not involve a linear relationship between theory and practice wherein the former determines the latter; rather it is a reflexive relationship in which both action and reflection build on one another. "The act of knowing involves a dialectical movement which goes from action to reflection and from reflection to new action" (Freire, 1972, p. 31). Through critical dialogue, people become "masters of their thinking by discussing the thinking and views of the world explicitly or implicitly manifest in their own suggestions and those of their comrades" (p. 95). Praxis, therefore, is constituted by both a theoretical and an experience component and is mediated by dialogue. As Wallerstein and Bernstein (1988) explain, "the goal of group dialogue is critical thinking by posing problems in such a way as to have participates uncover root causes of their place in society—the socio-economic, political cultural, and historical contexts of peoples lives" (p. 382). It is through this emancipatory dialogue that people are liberated to act in ways that enhance society. Conceptualizing the relationship between theory and practice this way reorients our thinking about pedagogy from searching for understanding and explanation to ethical action toward societal good (Hills & Mullett, 2000). This conceptualization is clearly embraced by nursings' Caring Science theory and philosophy.

AXIOLOGY

Heron and Reason argue that any inquiry paradigm also must consider a fourth factor—axiology. This factor is often overlooked in other paradigms, but it is essential to the participatory paradigm.

Axiology deals with the nature of value and captures the value question of what is intrinsically worthwhile? The fourth defining characteristic of an emancipatory relational pedagogy, axiology, highlights the "values of 'being', about what human states are to be valued, simply because of what they are" (Heron & Reason, 1997, p. 287). The participatory paradigm addresses this axiological question in terms of human flourishing. Human flourishing is viewed as a "process of social participation in which there is a mutually enabling balance, within and between people, of autonomy, co-operation and hierarchy. It is conceived as interdependent with the flourishing of the planet ecosystem" (Heron & Reason, 1997, p. 11). Human flourishing is valued as intrinsically worthwhile and participatory decision making and is seen as a means to an end "which enables people to be involved in the making of decisions, in every social context, which affect their flourishing in any way" (Heron, 1997, p. 11).

In this way, human flourishing is tied to practical knowing, knowing how to choose, how to be, and how to practice in ways that are not only personally fulfilling but that also enhance and transform the human condition. This concept of human flourishing is similar to Friere's (1987) notion of conscientization. As he explains, "Even when you individually feel yourself most free, if this is not a social feeling, if you are not able to use your freedom to help others to be free by transforming the totality of society, then you are only exercising an individualistic attitude towards empowerment and freedom" (p. 109). This valuing of human flourishing reconnects nurses to the human condition and recognizes the "truth" in our actions and practices. It means that in an emancipatory relational pedagogy, what is of interest is more than the usual educational outcomes. The utility of the educational outcome is judged based on the difference it makes to transforming the health and well-being of the society.

EMANCIPATORY RELATIONAL PEDAGOGY: INTERLOCKING CIRCLES

In the previous sections of this chapter, we have presented the educational theories that have influenced our pedagogy, described our conceptualization of pedagogy, and explored knowledge development from an emancipatory relational pedagogy. Now, in this final section of the chapter, we synthesize those conceptualizations and understandings into our framework for an emancipatory relational pedagogy for Caring Science curricula and introduce and describe the four elements that compose our framework for an emancipatory relational pedagogy.

We view the teaching-learning process as a relational inquiry because we believe that learning occurs in the relationship that is created by the teacher and learner and the knowledge that they create together. Knowledge is not something that the teacher has that is somehow transmitted to the learner. Nor is it something that the student discovers by her/himself, (although of course this can and does happen). We believe that learning actually occurs at the juncture of the authentic caring relationship that is created and lived by the teacher and students and the knowledge that they cocreate. Learning is a dynamic lived human experience.

An emancipatory relational pedagogy aims to create a relationship between teacher, learner, and knowledge that is based on a carefully edified thoughtfulness that attends to people's lived experiences and the meanings they create from those experiences. This notion of lived experience and its inherent concept of meaning making are at the heart of understanding emancipatory relational pedagogies. As vanManen (1990), explains "lived experience is the breathing of meaning" (p. 36). Dilthey suggested that "lived experience is to the soul what breath is to the body" (1985).

Transformational learning does not simply occur. In fact, we believe that four essential elements must be present and active for transformative learning to occur. They are: creating collaborative caring relationships, engaging in critical caring dialogue, reflecting-in-action, and creating a culture of caring. Each of these elements have underlying processes that drive the learning process. Each of the elements and their underlying processes are introduced here in this chapter and are described in detail in the chapters that comprise the remainder of this unit. Although we describe them separately, they work in synergy and, together, they represent our conceptualization of an emancipatory relational pedagogy.

Creating Collaborative Caring Relationships

The first essential component of an emancipatory relational pedagogy is creating collaborative relationships. In our own teaching, we are committed to fostering egalitarian teaching/learning relationships based on trust, caring, mutual respect, and shared power. We believe that, for learning to occur, all involved must feel safe, trust each other, and be committed to the process in which they are engaged. Collaborative caring relationships need time to develop and usually require several mutual experiences with positive outcomes. Collaborative caring relationships usually result in a synergistic alliance of the participants, an alliance with one another and with the knowledge that is cocreated. This element is described and discussed fully in Chapter 4.

Engaging in Critical Caring Dialogue

For us, critical dialogue is the touchstone of an emancipatory relational pedagogy. When it is done well, it encourages critical thinking, critical reflection, the creation of new knowledge, and the discovery of personal meaning. It draws upon original thinking, unique personal interpretations, inner wisdom, and subjective life experiences. It is often the most difficult aspect of a teaching/learning experience because it requires that we challenge our own and others' assumptions, engage in healthy debate, and be caring and respectful of each other, all at the same time. We believe deeply and passionately that people are able and that our responsibility as teachers is to create ambiguity, to challenge taken-for-granted assumptions, and to create an environment in which learners feel free to wrestle with ideas, challenge us and other learners, share half-baked ideas, and engage in critical dialogue about the issues at hand. During and after a critical dialogue, one should feel invigorated, thoughtful and, at times, exhausted. Feelings of pondering and exhilaration occur simultaneously. Most important, at the end of this kind of dialogue you should feel that your ideas were challenged but that your self-esteem and your caring relationship are intact! The second component, engaging in critical caring dialogue, is explored in Chapter 5.

Reflection-in-Action

The third component of an emancipatory relational pedagogy is reflection-in-action. Reflection-in-action emphasizes the importance of having actual reflective, mindful experiences, integrated with knowledge development and learning. Reflection-in-action attends to the development of mindfulness, of catching oneself in the moment in learning, processing, of critiquing oneself. It is related to becoming a silent witness to your own feelings, thinking, and knowing. This process is related to how to mindfully take action and do something rather than merely being able to talk about how something should or could be done.

To be able to maximize reflection-in-action, we must be prepared to be self-aware in the moment: to be able to reflect in the midst of acting, being open to changes in thinking and practice, in our actions. Self-awareness and evolving consciousness of our own behavior in the moment is critical to our ability to be reflective and to develop insight. It involves self-correction on the spot in our actions, behaviors, and practices with ourselves and with others. This ability is generated from being intentional and conscious of both one's self and others—in the-moment. A critical caring environment within an emancipatory relation pedagogy reinforces safety of self-critique, and feedback allows one to examine our inner most concerns, doubts, questions, and queries, and, most importantly, express them. This process nurtures our development as a learner and teacher; it fosters personal/professional growth and deepens our connection and abilities to further own evolution and inner knowing. This third component is explored in Chapter 6.

Creating a Culture of Caring

The final component, creating a culture of caring, is covered in Chapter 7. This surrounds and encapsulates the other three elements of our emancipatory relational framework (Figure 3.2).

We must acknowledge our nursing culture—it exists. We have all experienced it in our work places or even when we meet other nurses in social situations. We have a way of talking, being with, and relating to one another and a *shortcut way* of engaging with each other because we share this culture, the culture of nursing. Our culture includes our values, taken for granted assumptions, traditions, our way of doing things, and our ways of relating to each other and others. It can be subtle or sometimes not it, but it does exist.

As nurse educators working within a Caring Science curriculum, we need to include as part of our emancipatory pedagogy a deliberate effort to create a culture of caring in a way that transcends education and becomes a conscious, articulated way of practicing nursing. This requires more than simply creating a safe environment for learning. It means embracing a caring stance and being caring in our relationships with students and peers and colleagues so that we demonstrate how to enact our caring culture. Caring is not a soft and warm feeling; it is a moral obligation to act ethically and justly. In order to cultivate this caring way of being, nurse educators need to provide precedence for this caring culture over the more traditional bio-medical/technocure culture that has been so dominant in nursing and nursing education. In order to cultivate this caring way of being, nurse educators need to provide precedence for this caring culture over the more traditional bio-medical/technocure culture that has been so dominant in nursing and nursing education. The precedence of this caring culture is the true reflection of the nature of nurse-client and teacher–student relationships, and it is within this context that nurses must be educated if we are to fulfill our mandate to society. As caring science nurse educators we are obligated to attend to this development. This element is explored more fully in Chapter 7.

The following diagram represents the interrelationship of the four key elements (Figure 3.3).

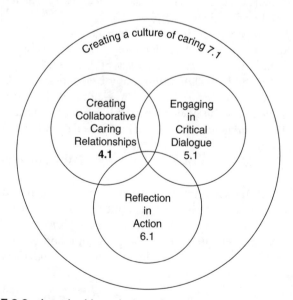

FIGURE 3.3 Interlocking circles of a caring science curriculum.

REFERENCES

Abram, D. (1996). *The spell of the sensuous: Perception and language in a more than human world*. New York: Pantheon.

Belinky, M. Clinchy, B., Goldenberger, N., & Tarule, J. (1986). *Women's ways of knowing*. Boston: Perseus Books Group.

Bevis, E., & Watson, J. (1989). Illuminating the issues: Probing the past, a history of nursing curriculum development—the past shapes the future. In E. Bevis & J. Watson (Eds.), *Toward a caring curriculum: A new pedagogy for nursing*. New York: National League of Nursing.

Carper, B. (1978). Fundamental patterns of knowing in nursing. *Advances in Nursing Science, 1*(1), 13–23.

Chinn, P. (1989). *Feminist pedagogy in nursing education. Curriculum revolution: Reconceptualizing nursing education*. New York: National League for Nursing.

Combs, A. W. (1982). *A personal approach to teaching: beliefs that make a difference*. Boston: Allyn and Bacon.

Dilthey, W. (1985). *Introduction to the Human Sciences*. Boston: Princeton University Press.

Freire, P. (1972). *Pedagogy of the oppressed*. New York: Continuum.

Gore, J. (1993). *The struggle for pedagogies: Critical and feminist discourses as regimes of truth*. New York: Routledge.

Guba, E., & Lincoln, Y. (1994). Competing paradigms in qualitative research. In N. K. Denzin & Y. S. Lincoln (Eds.), *Handbook of Qualitative Research* (pp. 105–117). London: Sage.

Heron, J. (1997). *Cooperative inquiry*. London: Sage.

Heron, J., & Reason, P. (1997). A participatory inquiry paradigm. A participatory inquiry paradigm. *Qualitative Inquiry, 3*(3), 274–294.

Hills, M., & Mullett, J. (2000). Community-based research: Collaborative action for health and social change. In Victoria B. C. (Ed.), *Community Health Promotion Coalition*. Victoria BC: University of Victoria.

hooks, B. (1994). *Teaching to transgress: Education as the practice of freedom*. New York: Routledge.

Husserl, (1964). *Field of consciousness*. Pittsburgh, PA: Dusquesne University Press.

Ironside, P. M. (2001). Creating a research base for nursing education: An interpretive review of conventional, critical, feminist, postmodern, and phenomenologic pedagogies. *Advances in Nursing Science, 23*(3), 72–87.

Kenway, J., & Modra, H. (1992). Feminist pedagogy and emancipatory possibilities. In C. Luke & J. Gore (Eds.), *Feminisms and Critical Pedagogy* (pp. 138–167). New York: Routledge.

Lewin, K. (1947). Frontiers in group dynamics: Concept method and reality in social science: Social equilibria and social change. *Human Relations, 1*(1), 5–41.

Merleau-Ponty, M. (1962). *Phenomenology of perception.* New York: Taylor & Francis.

Polkinghorne, D. (1988). *Narrative knowing and the human sciences.* Albany, NY: State University of New York.

Rogers, C. (1969). *Freedom to learn: A view of what education might become.* (1st ed.). Columbus, OH: Charles Merrill.

Reason, P. (1988). *Human inquiry in action.* London: Sage.

Skolimowski, H. (1994). *The participatory mind: A new theory of knowledge and of the universe.* London: Penguin Books.

Schratz, M., & Walker, R. (1995). *Research as social change.* London: Sage.

van Manen, M. (1990). *Researching lived experience.* London, ON: Althouse Press.

Wallerstein, N., & Bernstein, E. (1988). Empowerment education: Freire's ideas adapted to health education. *Health Education & Behavior, 15*(4), 379–394.

Watson, J. (2000). Transformative thinking and a caring curriculum. In E. O. Bevis & J. Watson (Eds.), *Towards a caring curriculum: A new pedagogy for nursing* (pp. 51–60). Sudbury, MA: Jones and Bartlett.

4
Creating Caring Relationships: Collaboration, Power, and Participation

A real humanist can be identified more by his trust in the people,
which engages him in their struggle, than by a thousand actions
in their favor without that trust.
—Freire, 1972, p. 36

T HE PURPOSE OF THIS CHAPTER is to explore the first component
of an emancipatory relational pedagogy—creating caring relationships and to develop an understanding of how to create
such relationships. This chapter examines the three elements involved
in creating caring relationships: collaboration, power/empowerment,
and participation. These elements are essential to the development
of caring relationships (Figure 4.1).

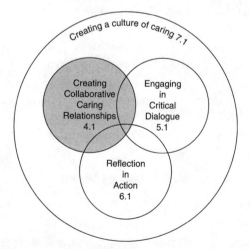

FIGURE 4.1 Interlocking circles of a caring science curriculum.

COLLABORATION: BEING-IN-RELATION

Throughout the literature and within scholarly debates about emancipatory relational pedagogies, there is agreement that, for significant learning to occur, the creation of collaborative, or what is often referred to as egalitarian, relationships is essential. But the literature and debates too often lack discussion about how to create such a relationship.

We live immersed in relationships of all sorts. We have our relationship to our self, to others (family members, colleagues, friends), and to society and the world. These relationships vary and have different characteristics, but we are always in relation even when we are alone. Further, we have a choice about how to be in those relationships, and we choose and change constantly in those relationships even though the dynamics of the relationship may try to keep it the same. It is also true that in nursing and nursing education, we choose how to be in relation to our patients/clients and our students. However, when you choose to embrace a Caring Science or emancipatory relational pedagogy, you are committing to developing a particular type of relationship with your patients and students. You are committing to developing a collaborative caring relationship.

What Is Collaboration?

The notion of collaboration can mean different things to different people. So, what does it mean to collaborate?

Time Out for Reflection

In your journal, respond to the following questions:

- What does it mean to collaborate?
- What is the difference between cooperation and collaboration, partnerships?
- How is power related to collaboration?
- What needs to be present in order for you to feel that you are engaged in a collaboration?
- What is your responsibility in contributing to this collaboration?

Collaboration has several definitions. In Webster's Dictionary, the first reads: "To work together as in a joint intellectual effort." Directly below this is a second definition: "To co-operate reasonably as with an enemy occupying one's country."

We believe this second definition captures a tension that can exist in collaborative relationships. When people who must work together (e.g., teachers and students; nurses and patients) view themselves as having different vested interests, each may feel like she/he has to protect her/his own "turf." We have all experienced situations in which we are trying to get someone to do something that we want to have happen, and they are not as invested in the same agenda and a certain tension results. The secret to overcoming this tension lies in finding a common vision: in cocreating what you each will work toward and how you will get there. This process for engagement needs to be transparent and agreed upon by teachers and students and/or nurses and patients.

For us, the following definition best describes the caring collaborative relationship that we try to create within an emancipatory relational pedagogy.

> Collaboration is the creation of a synergistic alliance that honours and utilizes each person's contribution in order to create collective wisdom and collective action. Collaboration is not synonymous with co-operation, partnership, participation or compromise. Those words do not convey the fundamental importance of being in relationship nor the depth of caring and commitment that is needed to create the kind of reciprocity that is collaboration. Collaborators are committed to, care about and trust in each other. They recognize that, despite their differences, each has unique and valuable knowledge, perspectives and experiences to contribute to the collaboration.

Being Collaborative

Collaboration demands that teachers relate person to person with their students. It is not possible to develop a relationship with someone who hides behind a role or is not fully present in some way. So the key responsibility of the teacher is to show up! Being present in a relationship requires a teacher to relate in ways that communicate deep caring for the student and a recognition of the student as a person of

Time Out for Reflection

In your journal . . .

- Review the key elements that you identified as being necessary for a collaborative relationship. Note how they compare to those elements outlined in the above definition.

- Recall a time when you felt you were participating in a collaborative relationship within a teaching/learning situation.

What was it about the situation that made it collaborative?

In your journal . . .

- List what you consider to be the key elements of a collaborative caring relationship.

worth, simply because she/he exists. As one faculty member, who was attempting to shift from a behavioral evaluation method to one that embraced a Caring Science paradigm explains, "our conversations and her journal allow me to see her [student] as a human being, a person seen in a holistic way; someone on a journey with her own way of knowing and understanding. The relationship with my past students was much more superficial; one based on a technical objective way of understanding . . . the old progress notes which constantly reflected the objectives seemed to keep us on task—the task of 'caring for people' who had a disease." "Taking care tended to be doing something *to* someone rather than *being* with someone" (Hills, 2000, p. 13)

In order to be able to develop relationships with students that embrace their humanity and personhood, teachers, first, must learn to be aware of and to care for themselves (Britzman, 1992).

LEARNING ACTIVITY:
RELATIONSHIPS ARE PERSONAL

Ends in View

The purpose of this learning activity is to examine the essential nature of a collaborative partnership as a personal commitment.

Write

In your journal, write five strategies that you could use to keep yourself in tune with how others perceive you. Reflect on the process you use to screen this information. How do you know the feedback someone gives you is "accurate"? How do you decide which information to act on? What strategies do you use to care for yourself? List five.

Share your responses to the above questions with a classmate.

Reflect

Do you have any concerns about relating in a personal way to students? In your journal, reflect on any such concerns. Set two goals that you can work on during this course that will assist you in developing this aspect of creating collaborative caring relationships.

Developing your "self," becoming all you can be, is one of the greatest gifts a teacher can give to others. Buscaglia (1982) argues that only through actualizing your *self* as a person do you have something to give to others. In short, you can't give what you don't have. "The most wondrous part of developing your self is that you can give it away and you don't lose anything by giving your self to others" (1982). Buscaglia encourages teachers to develop their uniqueness so that they can celebrate their humanness and have more to share with others:

> It all starts with you . . . If I grow and grow, I can give you more of me. I learn so that I can teach you more. I strive for wisdom so that I can encourage your truth. I become more aware and sensitive so that I can better accept your sensitivity and awareness. And I struggle to understand my humanness so that I can understand you when you reveal to me that you are only human too. And I live in continual wonder of life, so that I can allow you too to celebrate your life. What I do for me, I do for you. (p. 50)

Partners in Learning and Teaching

In creating caring relationships as part of an emancipatory relational pedagogy, teachers and students must be partners in the learning process. A "promotion" of learner-to-partner status is not the same as self-directed or student-centered learning. Self-directed and student-centered learning places the majority of the effort or work of learning on the learner. In emancipatory relational pedagogy, based on Caring Science, the work of learning is shared between teacher and learner. This idea may seem self-evident, but it is fundamental to the pedagogy that you develop. Teaching/learning practice looks very different within the different approaches. An emancipatory relational pedagogy is fundamentally a situation where the teachers and students both have to be learners, and both have to be cognitive subjects, in spite of them being different. For us, the first principle of an emancipatory relational pedagogy is for teachers and students to be critical agents in the act of knowing. As you are a teacher, so are you a learner. Every time you enter a situation with another for the purpose of engaging in an educational encounter, you simultaneously learn and teach. We are not suggesting that "teaching" is neutral or that how we are as teachers does not impact on the learning experience. Instead, we are trying to honor the importance of the cocreation of knowledge, when teachers and learners fully engage as passionate soul mates in their quest for deeper understandings. We believe this to be true no matter what the setting. So, for example, when you enter a learning situation with clients, as a nurse you would approach the situation not as much to "teach" clients about some aspect of their health but to engage with them in a caring relationship in which you cocreate mutually understood meanings about their situation; about their health and healing experience. All too often we hear teachers in teaching/learning situations say, "Well I gave them the information. I don't know what the problem is." Combs (1982) states that there are two faulty assumptions about teaching/learning that we must constantly guard against. The first is "If I taught it, it was learned"; the second is "We are not learning unless we are getting new information" (p. 45). But we know that learning has more to do with the *meaning* we make of the information than the actual transmission of that information. Information is not knowledge. So in situations with nurses and clients, as with nurse educators and students, it is imperative that we ascertain the meaning that is being made of the information that we are sharing. We do that by being in relationship and a partnership of learning/teaching.

LEARNING ACTIVITY

Write

In your journal, write about a teaching/learning situation in which you felt that you were a partner in the learning process. Consider and answer the following questions:

What was it about the situation that made it a partnership?

How was the partnership established?

How did the relationship, being a partnership, affect you and the teaching/learning process?

Dialogue

Share your experiences with your learning partners or study group. Discuss how your experiences are similar to or different from each other.

Reflect

In your journal, describe what you consider to be the essential characteristics of developing partnerships in teaching/learning situations.

POWER AND EMPOWERMENT

In this section, we explore the issue of power and discuss strategies for negotiating power while creating collaborative relationships. In addition, we discuss the concept of empowerment and its impact on the teaching/learning partnership.

The Pressure of Power

From an emancipatory relational pedagogy perspective, it is not possible to talk about pedagogy without talking about power. In fact, some pedagogies within this emancipatory perspective suggest that power is the key element upon which to focus (Friere, 1972; hooks, 1994). Others recognize power as important but tend not to deal as directly with it.

Because of the influence of Freire (1972) and hooks (1994) on our work, we view power as one of the most critical and pivotal concepts in any teaching/learning situation. Freire contends that if teachers and learners seized the power available to them in the classroom, they could remake society.

Power dynamics exist in all teaching/learning situations and, with each situation, there is a choice to be made about how power will be negotiated. You can choose to have *power over* others or you can choose to have *power with* others. Empowering relationships are characterized by power with partnerships that encourage full participation by all participants. Power lies at the centre of empowerment and "the empowering act exists only as a relational act of power taken and given in the same instance" (Labonte, 1990, p. 49).

In many situations it is not possible to have *equal* power. For example, in a formal teaching/learning situation such as in a nursing course in a nursing program, the teacher has responsibility to grade the students' assignments. Imagine that we are teaching you in such a course. We are automatically given power over students, but we can decide how to use that power. We can negotiate power but, in all of our years of teaching, we have not found a system that allows an equal distribution of power around this issue of grading. However, we can and possibly should be transparent about the process, negotiate the criteria, and include peer and self-critique in the assessment of your work. An exemplar of such an approach is discussed in Chapter 13. You always have the choice to offer alternatives and to negotiate other options. "At its simplest, power is about choice" (Labonte, 1990, p. 50).

Time Out for Reflection—Examining Your Experiences

Think about a time when you were in a teaching/learning situation that felt empowering. In your journal, identify what the key factors were that made you feel you had control.

- Was there a power differential in this situation?

- How was power negotiated in this situation?

- What strategies were used to encourage "power sharing"?

- What strategies will you use to encourage students to share power?

Nurses often face issues of power when talking about other people's health issues. Nurses are familiar with labeling others' problems with medical terminology and reporting on others' progress using nursing or medical jargon, so it is sometimes difficult to let clients or students tell their story without similarly labeling their issue. Clients/ students are much more likely to describe their (health) concern in relation to their lived experience of it than to label it as a medical diagnosis. Naming our own experiences is powerful in and of itself. "Our first claim to power—power being defined as the capacity to create or resist change—is naming our experiences and having that naming heard and respected" (Labonte, 1997, p. 31). In order to create collaborative relationships that are empowering, clients or students must name and describe the (health) issue or experience. "The ability to tell one's story, and to have access to and influence over collective stories, is a powerful resource" (Rappaport, 1995, p. 802).

One teaching strategy that was used in a Caring Science curriculum (Hills, 1994) was to teach students to learn about patient's health and healing experiences by learning about the patient's story. One student, reflecting on her experience states:

> My client is a good teacher. She openly explained the physiological factors of Parkinson's disease, her past history with the disease, and what her experiences had been like for herself, and how it has affected various members of her family. . . . So far, I haven't been in a position to teach my client much. I've basically been learning from her. I feel good bout this method of learning—no textbook could have told me this resident's personal story. (p. 8)

Nursing has been reluctant to trust people to act in their own best interests; "on the whole, professionals do not trust ordinary people, seeing them as lacking knowledge living inappropriate lifestyles, absconding with resources and generally not doing what they should to keep themselves healthy" (Raeburn & Rootman, 1999, p. 19). If we want to change this undermining of people/clients, nurse educators must develop teaching strategies that are empowering of students so that they in turn can empower their clients. Students can't empower others, if they don't experience empowerment themselves. The following learning activity provides typical nursing situations that provide opportunities to practice empowering responses.

LEARNING ACTIVITY:
Naming Health Problems

Ends in View

In this learning activity, you will examine power in relation to naming health issues and problems. When working with clients in teaching/learning situations, encouraging individuals or groups to name their health issue is one of the fundamental principles of creating a caring relationship.

Consider the Following Scenarios:

Scenario 1: You are a public health nurse doing a follow-up antenatal visit with a first-time mother. There were no complications with the birth, and you are expecting a routine visit. When you enter the home, you are greeted by a tired mother, who reports she has been up half the night and feels like she hasn't slept in days. She tells you that she feels like shaking the baby to make him stop fussing and asks you what you know about colic.

Scenario 2: You are a hospital nurse and you have been caring for Johnny, who has been admitted for the third time in 6 months with asthma. You have been doing discharge teaching with his mother, who is divorced and on social assistance. You have had several discussions with her about the importance of keeping the home as dust free as possible and of Johnny avoiding smoke or other pollutants. On the day before Johnny is to be discharged, his mother approaches you and says that she needs to speak to you about something important. You find a quiet place to sit, and she begins the conversation by telling you that she smokes.

Write

In your journal, write two responses to each of these scenarios. In the first, describe a way of responding that is NOT empowering, in which you, as the nurse, name what is happening. In the second, describe how you might respond in a way that is empowering and that encourages the client to name her health issue.

Dialogue

With your group, take turns sharing and critiquing each other's responses. Discuss how it might feel to be the recipient of the different responses (the client/learner). Did the empowering responses feel different than when the nurse was naming the health issue?

Reflect

In your journal, identify strategies you could use to encourage clients to name their health issue or concern. How can you encourage clients to share their health experiences and stories?

PARTICIPATION

The third element, essential to creating collaborative caring relationships, is participation. Having full participation in a teaching/learning situation is not always easy. Students and teachers enter classrooms or clinical areas already consumed by daily life. Em Bevis used to comment that when you arrive somewhere different or new, you need to give your soul time to catch up to your body. This type of centering or preparing to be present is critical for participation to occur within an emancipatory relational pedagogy. In this section, we describe participation and suggest strategies for encouraging participation.

Participation Versus Involvement

Without participation, there can be no partnership or relationship. Participation is a slippery concept and is often confused with the notion of involvement. In the realm of community development, Labonte (1997) has conceptualized some interesting distinctions between these two terms. We have adapted his conceptualization for our emancipatory relational pedagogy. In this context, the following distinctions are important:

Characteristics of Participation

- negotiated, formalized relationships
- open frame of "problem-naming"
- shared decision-making authority
- teacher/learner fully recognized as partners in learning
- shared responsibility and accountability for learning/teaching
- power is negotiated

Characteristics of Involvement

- learners are asked opinions that may or may not be used
- some sharing of power but ultimate authority rests with teacher
- decision making rests with teacher
- power remains with teacher; students asked to contribute ideas

Considering the distinctions presented above, we can see that participation is very different than merely being involved. Participation requires commitment. It is a conscious decision to devote time, energy, and resources to teaching/learning. Participation demands engagement.

LEARNING ACTIVITY:
PARTICIPATION OR INVOLVEMENT: WHAT SHALL IT BE?

The purpose of this learning activity is to examine your experiences of participation and involvement so that you can discover strategies for participation.

Write

Describe a teaching/learning situation in which you felt that participation was present. Use the above criteria to list the critical elements that made it a situation of participation rather than one of involvement.

How do you see these two terms?
How are they related to each other?
Think about strategies you can use to ensure you have participation in teaching/learning situations.

Reflect

In your journal, list five strategies you can use to ensure participation. Describe any concerns you have about encouraging participation. Write down three of your strengths that will assist you to encourage participation.

In her book, *Peace and Power*, Peggy Chinn (2008) describes several strategies for creating full group participation that rely on power with relationships: strategies that she refers to as "peace" processes. She suggests the following guidelines for encouraging participation:

- Give every perspective full voice.
- Demystify all processes and structures.
- Fully respect different points of view.
- Pay attention to the process itself so that how you do things is just as important as what you do.
- Rotate and share leadership according to ability and willingness.
- Value learning new skills so that the opportunity is accessible to all.
- Share responsibility for the processes of the group equally among everyone present.

As teachers, we each need to find our own ways to foster participation. There is no golden rule that works for everyone in every situation. However, following the guidelines above will create opportunities for participation that might not otherwise exist.

One way of implementing Chinn's recommendations for encouraging participation is to develop group guidelines for discussion. This not only demystifies the group process and encourages participation but it also creates solidarity between teachers and students resulting in joint responsibility and accountability for learning and teaching.

Developing Guidelines for Discussion

Many teaching/learning situations occurring in groups or group work is often incorporated in teaching/learning situations where the group is too large to function as a whole. Whether you are working with a large or small group, within an emancipatory relational pedagogy group discussion is a favored teaching strategy. Many years ago, Combs (1965) made an important distinction between group participation for the exploration of purposes and group participation for decision making. Confusing these types of discussion and participation can lead to difficult group dynamics. Most learning groups are developed for the purpose of exploration. That is, they are used to engage students in critical thinking and critical dialogue for the purpose of learning.

Group Participation for Exploration

We find it useful when teaching in group or using group dialogue to clarify the purpose of group and to establish guidelines for participation. We usually begin by sharing some of our own and having students add, change, modify them to make them unique for this particular group. The following are guidelines that we have created that we ask students to discuss and then create their own.

Guidelines for participation for Exploration (adapted from Combs 1965)

- Maintain an attitude of searching for understanding and meaning. Try to let go of previously held ideas so that they don't interfere with your ability to think creatively.
- Share your "half-baked" ideas. They are often more interesting than what you already know.
- Stay in a state of not knowing. It is only when you don't know something that you can learn. If you already know something, there is no need to explore it.
- Cultivate the art of empathic listening. Try to synthesize or summarize what others have said before your make your contribution.
- Stay with the group. Follow the trend of the discussion and introduce new topics when old ones are complete.

- Talk briefly. Saying too much may cause others' minds to wander and then they may miss what you wish to express.
- When you disagree, be respectful. You can be challenging without being confrontational.

In addition to the guidelines described above, it is often helpful to ask groups to establish their own guidelines by asking "What needs to happen for you to feel safe to explore your ideas?" Students and teachers can then together create their ground rules for participation in the learning/teaching environment.

Time Out for Reflection

Think of different strategies you could use to establish patterns of working together in groups that enhance participation. How would you deal with students who are silent in the group? How will you deal with students who talk too much in the group? How will you ensure that the ground rules are honored? Who is responsible for maintaining collaborative relationship?

Reflect

In your journal, list two strategies you could use for establishing group norms that are consistent with the ones outlined above. How will you ensure that the cocreated group norms will be honored in your emancipatory relational pedagogy?

In any teaching/learning situation, it is imperative to make the process for discussion and decision making transparent. Using a learning activity, such as the one you just completed, is one way of ensuring that this process occurs. There are many other ways to accomplish this goal. You need to discover what will work best for you. In situations involving individuals, the same process needs to occur, but it is usually done through one-on-one dialogue rather than a learning activity.

LEARNING ACTIVITY:
CHECKING IN AND CHECKING OUT

Ends-in-view

The purpose of this learning activity is to provide opportunities for you to experiment with two strategies for encouraging ongoing collaborative partnerships.

Connecting as a Group

"Checking In" and "Checking Out" (Chinn, 2008) are useful strategies for continuously reminding the teaching/learning group of the collaborative nature of the group. These strategies also ensure that you hear from each group member, at least twice during a learning session. The most powerful aspect of these strategies is that it reminds learning groups of our individual humanity and humanness. When well facilitated, these strategies develop group cohesion and a sense of belonging.

Write

You have probably had experiences using these two strategies in other courses you have taken in your nursing program. In your journal, write about times when you used these strategies and they really seemed to work well.

- What occurred to make them work well?
- You probably have had experiences with these strategies that were not positive.
- What was it that didn't work?
- Describe your experiences. What needs to be in place for these strategies to work for you.

Reflect

In your journal, write about how you will take responsibility for ensuring that, if you use these strategies, they are working for people.

LEARNING ACTIVITY:
COLLABORATIVE DECISION MAKING

In this learning activity, you will have opportunities to develop strategies for collaborative decision making.

Group Decision Making

There may be times in a group when it is necessary to make decisions. How this process is handled must be congruent with the principles established for group process. For example, decisions may need to be made about negotiating for more time in a teaching/learning session, about a specific task that the group decides to take on, or about some point of controversy that the group stumbles upon. The point is that the decision-making process must support and be congruent with the group discussion process if you want to have collaborative relationships.

Groups often having difficulty coming to consensus on issues resort to voting as a way of being democratic. This strategy in fact can be coercive, and there are probably many other strategies that are more democratic. I have found the following strategy useful in my work with students. When we need to make a decision, we first have a full discussion so that everyone has an opportunity to share their views. A group member then states the issue and asks every member to give one of three responses: "I agree," "I disagree," or "I can live with it." If even one group member disagrees with the issue, further discussion is necessary.

Write

In your journal, write down five things that are important to you in group decision making.

Dialogue

Decide how you will make decisions collaboratively. Be sure to get full agreement from each member of the class about the process to be used. Each time you meet, clearly identify times when you need to make decisions and use the agreed-upon process to do so.

Reflect

In your journal, write down the collaborative decision-making process. Does it address the five issues that you wrote down earlier in your journal? If not, be sure to raise these issues at your next class.

REFERENCES

Britzman, D. (1992). The terrible problem of knowing thyself: Toward a poststructural account of teacher identity. *Journal of Curriculum Theorizing, 9*(3), 23–46.

Chinn, P. (2008). *Peace and power.* London: Jones Barlett.

Freire, P. (1972). *Pedagogy of the oppressed.* London: Penguin Books.

Labonte, R. (1990). *Empowerment practices for health professionals.* Toronto, ON: Participation.

Labonte, R. (1994). Health promotion and empowerment: Reflections on professional practice. *Health Education Quarterly, 21*(2), 253–268.

Labonte, R. (1997). *Power, partnerships and participation in health promotion practice.* Melbourne: Australia Press.

Rappaport, J. (1995). Empowerment meets narrative: Listening to stories and creating settings. *American Journal of Community Psychology, 23*(5), 795–897.

5
Engaging in Critical Caring Dialogue

*Education should have as one of its main tasks to invite people
to believe in themselves. It should invite people to believe they
have the knowledge.*
—Freire 1972, p. 80

I N THIS CHAPTER, WE PRESENT the second component of our emancipatory relational pedagogical framework—engaging in critical caring dialogue. The purpose of this chapter is to provide opportunities for you to examine the impact of engaging in critical dialogue as a fundamental element of emancipatory pedagogy (Figure 5.1). Critical dialogue consists of three essential interwoven

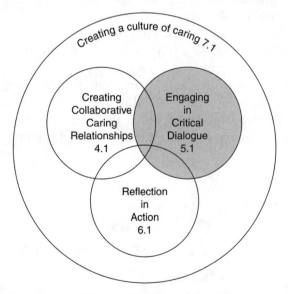

FIGURE 5.1   Interlocking circles of a caring science curriculum.

processes and elements: listening, critical questioning, and critical thinking. We will explore them in this chapter.

Critical dialogue is the backbone of an emancipatory relational pedagogy. It provides the answer to the *how* question. Dialogue might be considered simply a discussion, but critical dialogue is well planned, somewhat structured, and always purposive. The main purpose of critical dialogue is to create opportunities for critical thinking and critical reflection that result in the creation of new understandings (knowledge). Always transformative, critical dialogue aims to put teachers and students in situations where they *encounter* preconceived notions and ideas in ways that encourage them to question their assumptions. Without this type of encounter, they may be engaged in a discussion, but it would not be a critical caring dialogue.

LISTENING: THE HEART OF CRITICAL DIALOGUE

Listening is the most important process in critical caring dialogue, and it is the heart of an emancipatory relational curriculum. Without effective listening, dialogue is reduced to mere words. We can begin to engage in the critical caring dialogue only through understanding another's meaning.

The Chinese characters that represent the verb *to listen* reveal the complexity of listening (Figure 5.2). Listening involves seeing, hearing, and your heart.

There is magic in listening. Being able to hear another's issues and concerns with deep understanding is a rare gift. Effective listening requires a depth of caring about the other that is characterized by warmth, genuineness, and mutual respect. Listening requires an

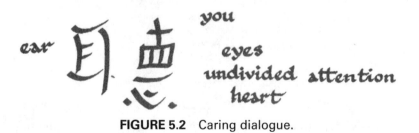

FIGURE 5.2 Caring dialogue.

ability to put aside, at least momentarily, our own thoughts and prejudices so that we can be open to the world of the other, so that we can be truly present with the other. Listening gives us access to the meanings that others are making in a given situation. Having this understanding of others permits us to respond in ways that are empathic and caring. Moustakas (1977) eloquently describes this process.

> Listening is a magnetic and strange thing, a creative force. . . . The friends that listen to us are the ones that we move toward, and we want to sit in their radius as though it did us good, like ultraviolet rays. . . . When we are listened to, it creates us, makes us unfold and expand. Ideas actually begin to grow in us and come to life. . . . It makes people happy and free when they are listened to. . . . When we listen to people, there is an alternating current, and that recharges us so that we never get tired of each other. We are constantly being recreated. (p. 32)

One of the most exciting things about this kind of listening, empathic listening, is that it can be learned. As Peavy (1972) explains, "It is not easy to listen well—it takes concentration, willingness and practice. For those who persist, the rewards are truly astounding" (p. ii).

Empathic listening requires not only that we hear what is being said but also that we respond in ways that demonstrate that we understood another's meaning. The acid test for empathic listening is not whether **we** think we have demonstrated this understanding but whether **the one being listened to** feels we have understood his/her meanings and experiences. Well-intentioned responses can often be misinterpreted as lack of understanding. This may be because, in general, we tend to judge ourselves by our intentions and others by their actions. For example, I might make what I intend to be a humorous comment; you might interpret that comment as sarcastic. I might say, "I was just trying to be funny!" but your interpretation can only be based on your observation and my action, not my intention. Others cannot access our thinking, so the only way they can interpret what we say or do is by our action, our response. That is how they will interpret how well we have understood them.

There are many different perspectives on the role of listening in teaching/learning. What Freire (1972) describes as listening for interests,

Rogers (1979) and Combs (1982) describe as empathic listening. Regardless of its description, there is no dispute about the significance of the role that listening plays in the teaching/learning process within an emancipatory relational pedagogy.

For us, the main difference between these conceptualizations of listening is not in how they are labeled but in the way that the theorists have viewed listening throughout their study of the teaching/learning process. For example, Rogers suggests that listening, coupled with respect and genuineness, is sufficient to bring about change. Freire argues that listening is important because it helps to identify the generative themes that need to be discussed through engagement in critical dialogue in order to move to action.

How does listening fit into your emancipatory relational pedagogical model?

LEARNING ACTIVITY:
LISTENING AND DEMONSTRATING UNDERSTANDING

Ends in View

This learning activity engages you in a role-play to illuminate critical aspects of empathic listening.

Dialogue

Part A

Have a discussion with your learning partner to decide on an issue that you both feel strongly about but upon which you disagree. This role-play will be most effective if you discover an issue that you really care about. If more than two people are involved, take turns in a one-on-one situation. Take a few minutes to quietly think about the issue. Think about the last time you discussed the issue with someone. Recall your feelings. When you are ready, each of you take 5 minutes to try to convince the other of the merits of your side of the issue. After your turn, take a few minutes to talk about how it felt to be involved in this type of discussion. Did you feel you were understood?

Part B

Find a token that you can easily pass between you (a pen or piece of paper). Continue your discussion, but this time with one difference. Only the person holding the token can state their opinion. The other must EARN the token by demonstrating that she/he has understood the other's perspective by responding empathically. Once you have earned the token, you may state your opinion, and the other person will try to earn it back by listening and responding empathically.

If you are the person with the token, do not give it up easily. The token must be earned by having your feeling understood. Remember not to confuse agreement with empathy. The purpose of this activity is to experience truly being heard even when the one who is hearing you does not agree with you.

Part C

Discuss your reaction to the role-play experience. How did the second experience differ from the first? In the second experience, did you experience feeling understood? If not, what would have made a difference?

Reflect

Write about your reactions to the above exercise. How did it feel to try to listen to someone with whom you disagreed? Describe your experience of listening empathically.

The following poem (anonymous) highlights the complexity and importance of listening for understanding in a way that demonstrates caring. Sometimes, when we try to be understanding, we unknowingly can be very unhelpful by giving advice, trying to solve the problem, telling people what they should do or feel, or negating their feelings. This poem identifies some of the ways we are tempted to respond when all that is desired by the other is to be heard and to feel cared for.

Listen

When I ask you to listen to me and you start giving me advice,
you have not done what I have asked.

When I ask you to listen to me
and you begin to tell me why I shouldn't feel that way,
you are trampling on my feelings

When I ask you to listen to me
and you feel that you have to do something to solve my problem,
you have failed me; strange as that may seem.

Listen! All I ask is that you listen,
not talk or do—just hear me.
Advice is cheap—10 cents will get you both Dear Abby
and Billy Graham in the same newspaper.

And I can do for myself; I'm not helpless
Maybe discouraged and faltering. But, not helpless.

When you do something for me that I can and need to do
for myself, you contribute to my fear and weakness.

But, when you accept as a simple fact that I do feel what I feel,
no matter how irrational,
then I can quit trying to convince you
and I can get about the business of understanding what's behind
this irrational feeling.

And when that's clear, the answers are obvious
and I don't need advice.
irrational feelings make sense when we understand.

Perhaps, that is why prayer works, sometimes, for some people,
because God is mute and he doesn't give you advice or try to fix things.
"They" just listen and let you work it out for yourself.

So, please, listen and just hear me.
And, if you want to talk, wait a minute for your turn;
and I'll listen to you.
Anonymous

When you choose to teach from an emancipatory relational pedagogy, you enter a unique and special caring relationship. Teachers working within this pedagogy join the students in "genuine encounters of caring and being cared for" (Noddings, 1984, p. 75). As Noddings (1984) explains, no enterprise or special function (e.g., the role of a teacher) can relieve teachers from their responsibility as *the one caring*. In professions where encounter is frequent (as in teaching/learning situations) and where the ethical ideal of the other (student) is necessarily involved, "I am first and foremost one caring and second an enactor of special functions" (Noddings, 1984, p. 77). As a teacher, I am, first, the one caring. This means that as a teacher, learning to listen with all your *being* and responding empathically is the key to being in relation in an emancipatory relational pedagogy.

CRITICAL QUESTIONING

In this section of the chapter, we describe Freire's conceptualization of problem posing as a strategy for critical dialogue, and we present a variety of other ways to use critical questioning to engage in critical dialogue.

Problem Posing

Freire's (1972) model of empowerment education describes a three-stage methodology consisting of listening, which we discussed in the previous section; participatory dialogue, which we will explore in this section; and action, which we will discuss in Chapter 6.

Freire proposes that the main strategy of empowerment (emancipatory) education, namely critical dialogue, requires us to engage, as a group, in a process of problem posing rather than a process of problem solving. Problem posing is different from problem solving because it does not seek immediate solutions to problems. Rather, generative themes arising from the listening phase are "codified" and posed as problematics to raise group consciousness about specific issues. Wallerstein and Hammes (1991) contend that this process recognizes the complexity and the time needed to create effective solutions to societal issues. "An effective code shows a problematic situation that is many sided, familiar to participants and open-ended without solutions" (Wallerstein & Bernstein, 1988, p. 383). Freire describes these as *generative themes* because they generate energy that motivates people to act.

Freire contends that, through a process of dialogue that reflects on the generative themes raised through listening, people become "masters of their thinking by discussing the thinking and views of the world explicitly or implicitly manifest in their own suggestions and those of their comrades" (p. 95). As Wallerstein and Bernstein explain: "The goal of group dialogue is critical thinking by posing problems in such a way as to have participants uncover root causes of their place in society—the socioeconomic, political, cultural, and historical contexts of personal lives". (p. 382)

Freire cautions that "the liberating educator has to be very aware that transformation is not just a question of methods and techniques" (p. 35). If that were the case, we could simply substitute one set of methods for another. "The question is in a different relationship to knowledge and to society" (Freire, p. 35).

Critical thinking about generative themes identified in the listening phase does not occur spontaneously. The teacher is responsible for guiding this critical dialogue process by using a 5-step questioning strategy that moves discussion from the personal to the social analysis and to the action level. People are asked (1) to describe what they see and feel, (2) as a group, to define the many levels of the issue, (3) to share similar experiences from their lives, (4) to question why this problem exists, and (5) to develop action plans to address the problem.

Wallerstein and Bernstein (1988) have created a questioning process for critical dialogue. They begin by using *triggers* to initiate dialogue. A trigger is a concrete, physical representation of a critical issue, generative theme, or obstacle that has arisen in the listening phase of empowerment education. For example, you might use a videotape, a role-play, a poem, or a story. In their description of developing learning activities, Bevis and Watson (1989) call this notion using *a hook*. A hook serves the same purpose. It grabs the student's interest and attention. It orients the student to the issue to be explored.

Wallerstein uses the acronym SHOWED to represent the different stages of this teaching/learning process, which is built on a questioning cycle of What? Why? So what? Now what?

S   See—What do I see here? How do we name this issue?

H   Happening—What is happening? What is really happening to this person, group, or community? These first two questions are the description stage during which the participants/students name the issue.

O   Our—How does this issue relate to our lives? How is my experience similar or different? How do I feel about the issue?

W   Why—Why does this issue occur? What are the social, cultural, economic, and political influences that contribute to this problem?

E   Empowered—How can we become empowered to deal with this issue?

D   Do—What can we do? What action steps can we take to act on the problem? These last two questions deal with the action-planning phase of the process.

We have adapted the following from Wallerstein and Bernstein's work.

The trigger should

- be based on a generative theme that you have listened for in a teaching/learning situation;
- portray the theme as a familiar issue, immediately recognizable by the participants/students;
- focus on one concern but contain historical, cultural, and social connections.

Time Out for Reflection

Think about a teaching/learning situation for which you have to prepare. Consider the following questions:

What might you use as trigger to engage learners?

How did SHOWED method of guiding critical reflection fit with your caring science pedagogy?

Using Critical Questions to Prompt Critical Dialogue

Learning to ask critical questions is the key strategy to having effective dialogue. A dialogue method "systematically invites students or audiences to think critically, to co-develop the session with the expert or teacher, and to construct peer relations instead of authority-dependent relations" (Freire, 1972, p. 41). Using a dialogical learning process encourages teachers to move beyond the traditional lecture method to a dialectal process of interaction. This shift from lecture to dialogical teaching/learning transfers the responsibility from teachers being solely responsible for creating learning experiences to shared responsibility for learning that promotes the creation of new knowledge and self-actualization for teachers and students (Clark, 2006).

Learners also must develop the strategy of asking critical questions. As Bevis (1989) suggest, "Teaching in its true form is helping students learn new ways of approaching ideas and examining things by helping them learn to ask the appropriate questions" (p. 242). They learn to do so but experiencing positive caring, yet critical questioning, in their own learning.

People who want to use a dialogue method often struggle with the issue of how to incorporate information-giving into this process. Indeed, there are some who feel that lecturing has no place in a dialogue method of teaching/learning. "Regardless of its strengths, lecturing is an oppressive teaching strategy. It is oppressive because, among other reasons, learners must listen to information filtered through someone else's perspective and value system" (Bevis, 1989, p. 240). One strategy that works within an emancipatory relational pedagogy is to ask students if they want to hear your (the teacher's) conceptualization or the way you have synthesized the knowledge from the literature. Lecturing can be engaging, but it is very dependent on the teacher's charisma. If lecturing seems warranted, be sure that students are included in the process. Combining "mini" lectures with discussion also assists in reducing "teacher talk." The more you move away from lecturing toward dialogical teaching strategies the more you are situated in an emancipatory relational pedagogy. In general, ask rather than tell.

Bevis (2000) identify a passive-to-active continuum and recommend several methods that assist in active learning. Their description of a learning episode is reminiscent of Freire's (1972) three-stage method described above. A "learning episode is a natural grouping of events in which students engage in the process of acquiring insights, seeing patterns, finding meanings and significance, seeking balance and wholeness and making judgments or developing skills" (p. 223). Bevis suggests that, for learning to occur, three stages—operation, information, and validation—must occur although they can occur in any order.

Operation Phase

The operation phase is an issue or a problem that is used to "hook" the students' interest. The teacher's ability to invoke reality in an imaginative way and to raise real and relevant questions that stimulate students' interest and motivation is the key ingredient of this aspect of the learning episode. The operational aspect of the learning episode is most effective when students are provided with structure regarding how much time to spend, what questions are to be answered, and then are left to struggle with their ideas in small groups.

Information Phase

The information phase is more passive and consists of the student acquiring data related to the issue or problem that was raised or will be raised in the operation phase depending on the sequencing of the phases. It is essential that the information that the student's are seeking is *needed* to "solve" the issue raised. "Active learning requires that the students be engaged with an issue or problem that require them to need information in order to solve the problem" (p. 225). If the students don't need the information, and the lack of information flows over into the dialogue that is typical of the operation phase, students will pool their ignorance, not their knowledge. The most common way to gain information is by reading, watching, or listening. Teachers need to use their imaginations to devise strategies for engagement that motivate students to want information. Some examples include watching a video clip, listening to a tape, reading an article, going on a scavenger hunt, or engaging in some other type of activity.

Validation Phase

The final phase of the learning episode, validation, is the testing aspect and it occurs in reality. In nursing, the validation phase often occurs in the clinical area. Validation allows students to see what they can do. This phase develops students' confidence. Simulations can help build competence but confidence only comes with reality validation.

LEARNING ACTIVITY:
ASKING CRITICAL QUESTIONS

Ends in View

There are many ways to engage in critical dialogue. In this learning activity, you will explore the use of critical questioning in relation to critical dialogue.

Read

Review, in this text, the SHOWED framework (Chapter 4), Bevis' description of the learning episode, and Freire's three-stage method for learning.

Write

In your journal, do a comparative analysis of Bevis and Watson's description of active learning, including the learning episode, and Wallerstein and Bernstein's SHOWED method. Identify the conceptual similarities and differences of these two models.

Does one model fit better than the other within your framework/model for teaching/learning practice?

Are there certain aspects of each that you would like to incorporate into your framework/model?

Dialogue

With your learning partners or study group, discuss your analysis of the two models. Discuss some of the scholarly modalities and educational heuristics identified by Bevis and Watson. Which of these will be helpful in developing your framework/model for teaching/learning practice?

Reflect

In your journal, revisit your framework/model for teaching/learning practice. Have you considered what methodology you will use in it? Revise your framework in ways that may now seem appropriate. Describe how your methodology is congruent with other aspects of it?

So, how can the teacher's information and knowledge be conveyed to learners? We would suggest that there is no problem with teachers sharing their ideas and concerns. On the contrary, it is irresponsible not to share. In fact, as just described above, sharing information when it is needed is an excellent way to share information. The critical consideration is **how** teachers should share their ideas. There are two key points involved here—timing and process. As Shor and Freire (1987) explain:

> The question is not "banking" lectures or no lectures, because traditional teachers will make reality opaque whether they lecture or lead discussions. A liberating teacher will illuminate reality even if he or she lectures. The question is the content and dynamism of the lecture, the approach to the object to be known. Does it critically reorient students to society? Does it animate their critical thinking or not? (p. 40)

If teachers begin sessions with lectures, there is an unstated assumption that what you have to say is more important than what students think about the topic or issue. This difficulty is related to the issue of power that was discussed in the previous chapters. Turning this process around by posing questions first and then sharing your ideas helps to reduce the power differential inherent in most teaching/learning situations. It must be stressed that it is the type of questions that you ask that is so important. Asking questions that require students to respond with memorized answers or "teacher knows the answer and you have to guess" is no different than lecturing. Asking questions that provoke learners to think in new and as yet undiscovered ways leads to insight and stimulates knowledge creation.

There are times when it is appropriate for teachers to share their synthesis of information. You might think of these as "mini raps" or "mini lectures." It is also important to remember that you, as teacher, have equal rights and responsibilities to be a full participant in the critical dialogue—sharing your views and learning from others. We have found the following strategies to be helpful when engaging in critical dialogue as a teacher.

- Share your ideas as opinions, not truths.
- Ask permission or ask for interest in hearing about what you know from the literature about the topic.
- Start a teaching/learning session by posing critical questions.

- Encourage students to work on issues in partnerships or small groups. Most students feel more comfortable *testing out their ideas* in a small group before sharing with a larger group.
- Create innovative ways of accessing learners' understandings from their group work (other than reporting back). One strategy is to ask learners to come up with one question that still remains unanswered for them that they would like the large group to consider.
- Watch for teachable moments. Teachable moments are spontaneous occasions when students ask a question or pose an issue in such a way as to signify a readiness to learn that is *urgent*. These moments are basically enactments of the famous saying "When a child stands in awe and mystery of a falling rose petal, then it's time to teach the law of gravity" (Zukav, 1980, p. 54).
- Learn to create and live with ambiguity. Being comfortable in a place of *unknowing* is a critical skill for a teacher who wants to practice from an emancipatory relational pedagogy. Students need space and time to struggle in that place of *not knowing* and teachers need to support their struggle without providing *their* answer to the issue or struggle.

CRITICAL THINKING

In this section of the chapter, we examine the role of critical thinking within an emancipatory relational pedagogy. Opportunities are provided for you to examine your critical thinking development and abilities.

What Is Critical Thinking?

Critical thinking is a process that requires that we continuously and critically question the assumptions that underlie our customary, habitual ways of acting and thinking. It involves much more than analytical, rational processing of information or analyzing information for logical fallacies. At its core, critical thinking requires that we question our assumptions as they are enacted in our daily lives. Meizerow (1990) states that this can be very demanding because admitting that our assumptions might be distorted, wrong, or contextually relative implies that the fabric of our personal and political existence might rest upon faulty foundations. Even considering this possibility is profoundly threatening. If our past lives have been lived within faulty assumptive worlds, we are faced with the question of whether we have to jettison our current relationships, work, and political commitments in favor of some more authentic ways of living, whatever they may be?. (p. 192)

Critical thinking is a productive and positive activity. Critical thinkers are totally engaged in and passionate about life circumstances. They see themselves as creators of life experiences and they exude a sense of vitality and hope. They are optimistic and see the potential that being "critical" offers. They are passionate and committed yet open and flexible.

Brookfield (1987) identifies five characteristics of critical thinking. Although we are using his headings here to describe critical thinkers, we have taken considerable poetic license in describing the attributes of critical thinkers.

Critical Thinking Is a Process, Not an Outcome

Critical thinkers are constantly in a state of becoming. They are consistently engaged in a process of wondering or of questioning assumptions. They are skeptical not only of universal truths but of simplistic explanations of any phenomena. Regardless of their own biases, they can always raise doubts about the way a situation is being viewed.

Manifestations of critical thinking vary according to the contexts in which they occur; there is no formula or *right* or *wrong* way to be a critical thinker. Critical thinkers vary enormously in terms of how they appear in everyday life. Sometimes they are more apparent to us because of the way they process information. It is easier to recognize the critical thinking abilities of those who externalize their thinking than it is to recognize those whose thinking is internal.

Critical Thinking Is Triggered by Positive as Well as Negative Events

Much of the literature describes critical thinking as being triggered by only negative events (Dobrzykowski, 1994). These negative events apparently cause people to question previously held assumptions about the way the world and the people in it work and relate to each other and this questioning prompts careful scrutiny of what were previously unquestioned views. However, it is just as reasonable to think that critical thinking can arise from joyous occasions in which our previously held assumptions are called into question.

Critical Thinking Is Emotive as Well as Rational

At times, critical thinking is presented as if it were removed from emotions and feelings. But emotions are in fact central to critical thinking. Questioning our unquestioned assumptions, our taken-for-granted values, and the way in which we live our lives touches on the core of our emotions and requires that we tune into our feelings.

Time Out for Reflection

In your journal, draw a line down the middle of a page. On the left-hand side of the page, list the five characteristics of critical thinkers. On the right-hand side, next to each characteristic, write at least two behaviors that you exhibit that you feel demonstrate this characteristic in the way you engage in teaching/learning situations. Would others recognize these characteristics in you?

List five strategies you could use to help others to develop critical-thinking characteristics.

Write about what seems new to you regarding the way you now view critical thinking. What stands out for you as being important or needing attention?

Essential Components of Critical Thinking

Brookfield (1993) identifies four essential components for critical thinking.

* *Identifying and challenging assumptions*—For us, the questions "How do you know that?", "Who told you that that is true?", and "Why does that have to be the case?" all challenge our taken-for-granted assumptions. So often, we wander through life accepting what seems, for us, to be the natural order of events. It is by asking, "Why must

this be so?" that we begin to uncover what is usually and naturally assumed to be so. Challenging assumptions is often difficult because many people would prefer that you not upset their equilibrium.

- *Challenging the influence of context*—Critical thinkers are aware that practices, structures, and actions are never context free. They are able to see the influence of the context on a particular situation and understand the dynamics that occur because of this context. It is as though they are tuned into the nuances of a situation. Because they understand the complexity of context, they can respond instantaneously to a given situation even though they may have never previously been in such a situation.

- *Imagining and exploring alternatives*—Critical thinkers are aware of many different ways of operating other than the one that seems most apparent. Although they understand that the context of a situation makes something appear to be the most obvious way of doing something, they also realize that, if the context were to shift slightly, something else could appear to be the most obvious thing to do.

- *Reflective skepticism*—Critical thinkers have a healthy optimism about being skeptics. They know that the best way of understanding a situation is to be critical and to raise questions about it. They are wary of quick-fix solutions. They are able to question practices that have existed for a long time because they recognize that, just because they have worked in the past, they may not be appropriate now. And, just because everyone else agrees with them, that doesn't make them right!

LEARNING ACTIVITY:
COMPONENTS OF CRITICAL THINKING

Ends in View

This learning activity is designed to have you examine your ability to think critically.

Write

In your journal, write the four components of critical thinking. Take a few minutes to think about yourself in a teaching/ learning situation. Beside each component, describe one experience that you have had in which you either experienced yourself or experienced someone else struggling with this component of critical thinking.

Dialogue

Describe these experiences you have written about in your journal to your learning partners or study group. Discuss how you felt as you struggled with these issues. Describe some of the main things you learned about critical thinking as a result of these experiences.

Reflect

In your journal, write about one area of critical thinking that you would like to work on. Identify three strategies you will use to help you work on this aspect for the remainder of the course.

Developing Critical Thinking

Many authors have described and theorized about the development of critical thinking. Brookfield (1993) has summarized others' thinking about it and suggests that the pattern of the development of critical thinking involves five phases.

TRIGGER EVENT

Some unexpected event occurs that results in inner feelings of discomfort or perplexity. Many theorists suggest that these events are often negative. We like to conceptualize this occurrence as creating ambiguity or confusion. We often tell students that part of our jobs as teachers is to create this ambiguity or confusion. For us, this is related to the issue that we raised earlier. We believe that you can't learn, or maybe we should say think critically, if you are in a state of *knowing*. Significant learning occurs when you are in a state of disease, or confusion. The brain is a wondrous organ for it will not allow you to stay in this state of disease. It will keep mulling around the confusion until you sort it out.

APPRAISAL

This is the period of self-scrutiny—the mulling around the issue—we describe above. During this phase, the issues and concerns are identified and clarified.

EXPLORATION

Having seen discrepancies or anomalies, new ways of explaining them begin to be explored in order to decrease the discomfort that is experienced. During this phase, new ways of thinking or acting are tested out that seem more congruent with the perceptions of what is happening in our lives. Abbs (1974) summarizes this phase as searching for new ways of doing things, new answers, new ways of organizing one's worldviews. For us, it is a time of possibility; a time for creating new ways of being-in-the world; a time for developing our caring capacities.

DEVELOPING ALTERNATIVE PERSPECTIVES

From these explorations, come new ways of thinking that begin to make sense for our current situations. This is a transitional phase during which the old is left behind, and new ways are embraced. New knowledge and skills are developed for the way you now wish to be.

INTEGRATION

Once you have decided on the worth, accuracy, and validity of your new ways of thinking and living, you begin to weave these "into the fabric of your lives" (Brookfield, 1993, p. 27). At this stage, you achieve some level of integration of the previously conflicting feelings or ideas. Meizerow (1990) describes this process as perspective transformation, whereas Boyd and Fales (1983) suggest that this is the "point at which people experience having learned, or having come to a satisfactory point of closure in relation to an issue" (p. 28).

Time Out for Reflection

Write in your journal about a time when you felt that you experienced the development of critical thinking as described above. Think about a problem you had to solve or a decision you had to make. Try to be specific in describing your experience in relation to the stages suggested by Brookfield.

Respond to the following questions:

- Did you experience all of these stages?

- Did some of the stages seem more important than others?

- Recall your assumptions and how they might have changed during the process.

- What alternatives did you consider?

- How did you evaluate the effectiveness of your choice of alternatives?

REFERENCES

Abbs, P. (1974). *Autobiography in education.* London: Heinemann Educational.

Bevis, E. (1989). Teaching and learning: A practical commentary. In E. Bevis & J. Watson (Eds.) (1989). *Toward a caring curriculum: A new pedagogy for nursing* (pp. 217–257). New York: National League for Nursing.

Bevis, E. O. (2000). Nursing curriculum as professional education: Some underlying theoretical models. In E. O. Bevis & J. Watson (Eds.), *Towards a caring curriculum: A new pedagogy for nursing* (pp. 67–107). New York: National League for Nursing.

Bevis, E. O. (2000). *Towards a caring curriculum: A new pedagogy for nursing.* New York: National League of Nursing.

Bevis, E., & Watson, J. (Eds.). (1989). *Toward a caring curriculum: A new pedagogy for nursing.* New York: National League for Nursing.

Boyd, E. M., & Fales, A. W. (1983). Reflective learning: Key to learning from experience. *Journal of Humanistic Psychology, 23*(2), 99–117.

Brookfield, S. (1987). *Developing critical thinkers.* San Francisco: Jossey-Bass.

Brookfield, S. (1993). On impostorship, cultural suicide, and other dangers: How nurses learn critical thinking. *The Journal of Continuing Education in Nursing, 24*(5), 197–205.

Clark, M. (2006). Action and reflection: Practice and theory in nursing. *Journal of Advanced Nursing, 11*(1), 3–11.

Combs, A. W. (1982). *Personal approach to teaching: Beliefs that make a difference.* Boston: Allyn & Bacon.

Dobrzykowski, T. (1994). Teaching strategies to promote critical thinking skills in nursing staff. *The Journal of Continuing Education in Nursing, 25*(6), 272–276.

Freire, P. (1972). *Pedagogy of the oppressed.* London: Penguin Books.

Meizerow, J. (1990). *Fostering critical reflection in adulthood.* San Francisco: Jossey-Bass.

Moustakas, C. (1977). *Creative life.* New York: Van Nostrand Reinhold.

Noddings, N. (1984). *Caring: A feminine approach to ethics and moral education.* Berkeley, CA: University of California Press.

Peavy, V. (1972). *The empathic workbook.* Victoria: University of Victoria.

Rogers, C. R. (1979). *Freedom to learn.* Columbus, OH: C.E. Merrill Pub. Co.

Shor, I., & Freire, R. (1987). *A pedagogy for liberation: Dialogues on transforming education.* Westport, CT: Bergin & Garvey.

Wallerstein, N., & Bernstein, E. (1988). Empowerment education: Freire's ideas adapted to health education. *Health Education Quarterly, 15*(4), 379–394.

Wallerstein, N., & Hammes, M. (1991). Problem-posing: A teaching strategy for improving the decision-making process. *Journal of Health Education, 22*, 250–253.

Zukav, G. (1980). *The seat of the soul.* Free Press.

6
Critical Reflection-in-Action (Praxis): Emancipatory Action

Even when you individually feel yourself most free, if this feeling is not a social feeling, if you are not able to use your recent freedom to help others to be free by transforming the totality of society, then you are exercising only an individualistic attitude towards empowerment and freedom . . . While individual empowerment, the feeling of being changed, is not enough concerning the transformation of the whole of society, it is absolutely necessary for the process of social transformation.
—Shor & Freire, 1987, p. 109

C RITICAL REFLECTION-IN-ACTION IS the third element of our emancipatory relational pedagogical framework. We assert that, in order to create transformational learning, students must be provided with actual experience in which they can discover reflecting and acting in the moment. We refer to this practical and applied application of knowledge from experience as *praxis*. We reach that goal at the end of the chapter. Beforehand, we explore the relationships between experience, reflection, and action. This process of reflection is recognized as an important aspect of learning. We examine the complexities of reflection by presenting different perspectives that help to distinguish reflection as an internal process and reflection as dialectic. It is reflection as a dialectic—reflection in action—that we argue is the key to transformational learning. Reflection **on** action can lead to change; reflection-**in**-action always leads to change (Figure 6.1).

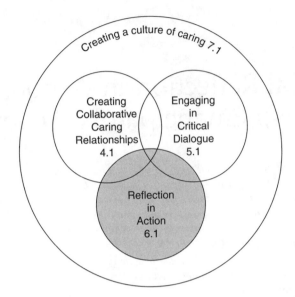

FIGURE 6.1 Interlocking circles of a caring science curriculum.

REFLECTION-ON-ACTION

Reflection is sometimes referred to as a process that occurs internally and in isolation. Boud (1985, pp. 18–40) states that "reflection in the context of learning is a generic term for those intellectual and affective activities in which individuals engage to explore their experiences in order to lead to new understandings and appreciations" (p. 19). Like Boud (pp. 18–40), Boyd and Fales (1983) also link reflection to experience and offer a useful definition of reflection as "the process of internally examining an issue of concern, triggered by an experience, which creates and clarifies meaning in terms of self, and which results in a changed conceptual perspective" (p. 100).

Reflection as a Three-Stage Process

Boud et al. have identified a three-stage process of reflection. They suggest that, in any learning experience, there are three stages—preparation, engagement, and processing, each of which require a different type of reflection. In the preparatory phase, learners deal with the anticipation of the experience, reflecting perhaps on what might be expected of them and what contribution they might make. In the engagement phase, the actual experience, students' reflections usually include recognition of the disparity between what they learned in the classroom and what they experience in the field. The final processing phase occurs after the field experience and involves retrospectively reflecting on the experience to make sense of it.

Assumptions Underlying Reflection in Learning

Boud et al. also detailed three key assumptions regarding reflection in learning:

- Only students themselves can learn and only they can reflect on their own experiences. Although, by a variety of methods, facilitators can access students' thoughts at a basic level, students have complete control in a teaching/learning situation by choosing what they are willing to share.
- Reflection is pursued with intent. It is a purposive activity directed toward a goal.
- Reflection is a complex process in which both feelings and cognition are closely interrelated and interactive.

LEARNING ACTIVITY:
REFLECTION ON OWN EXPERIENCES

Ends in View

In this learning activity, you will reflect on your own experiences and thoughts about reflection in learning.

Write

In your journal, write about a recent experience in which you felt that your learning was significant and meaningful. Address the following questions:
  What role did experience play in this situation?

How was reflection involved? Try to describe your process of reflection as concretely as possible.

What was the relationship between experience and reflection?

Dialogue

With your study group, discuss your responses to the above questions. Also, consider and discuss the following questions. How does reflection occur? What factors influence one's ability to reflect? How does one know that reflection has occurred?

Reflect

Review your journal entries in response to *learning activities* and/or time out for reflection activities that you have completed throughout this book. Pay particular attention to the notes that you have written for each reflection component of your numerous learning activities. Note any themes that seem to emerge. What characteristics of reflection seem evident?

Components of Reflection in Learning

Boud's (pp. 18–40) model for reflection in learning consists of two components—the experience and the reflective activity. They define experience as the total response of a person to a situation or event: what she/he "thinks, feels, does and concludes at the time and immediately thereafter" (p. 18). They contend that the experience is followed by a processing phase of reflection. Reflection is "an important human activity in which people recapture their experience, think about it, mull it over and evaluate it" (p. 19). In their view, one of the most important ways to enhance learning is to strengthen the link between experience and the reflective activity that follows it. It is recommended that teachers plan consciously for the reflective phase as it is often overlooked and undervalued.

Three elements were identified as being central to this reflective process (Boud et al., 1985):

1. *Returning to the experience*—This element involves recollecting the salient aspects of the experience. It is descriptive in nature and requires that the learner recall what actually occurred as accurately as possible. The simple recollection of an event can develop insight. As we witness the events again, they become available to us to reconsider and examine afresh; we realize "what we were feeling and what responses prompted us to act as we did" (p. 27). Boud (pp. 18–40) recommends that the description itself be as free from judgments and interpretations as possible.

2. *Attending to feelings*—This element involves the student consciously recalling positive and negative feelings that she/he may have encountered during the experience. Students are encouraged to use their own positive feelings to assist them in pursuing what otherwise might be a very challenging situation.

3. *Reevaluating the experience*—During this element, the experience is reexamined in light of the student's intent, while associating new knowledge with what was already known and integrating this new knowledge into the student's conceptual framework. Four aspects have been identified within this element of reevaluation (Boud, 1985):

    1. Association—Association is the connecting of the ideas and feelings that were a part of the original experience with those that have occurred during reflection. Through this process students may come to realize that their previous attitudes are no longer consistent with their new understandings.

    2. Integration—During this aspect of reevaluating the experience, the process of discrimination assists students in sorting out what is meaningful to them. Two processes are involved in this aspect: searching for the nature of relationships that have been observed in the association aspect and drawing conclusions while arriving at insights. The student experiences a coming together or creative synthesis of the information previously taken in and the formation of a new solution or change in the self—what might be called a new gestalt (Boyd & Fales, 1983, p. 32).

3. Validation—In this aspect, learners begin to test their new understandings for consistency with their existing knowledge and beliefs. If discrepancies appear, the situation needs to be reassessed in order to decide on what basis to proceed. Rehearsal is a useful strategy to use in the validation aspect.

4. Appropriation—This aspect does not occur in all instances of reevaluating the experience. This aspect involves the student owning the new information in a personal way. Strong emotions are involved in this process and the student often is affected deeply by the learning. The inclusion of the emotional quality to information radically alters the way that information is treated by the student's consciousness as they experience the personal meaning of the experience.

REFLECTION-IN-ACTION

Some theorists make a distinction between reflection-on action and reflection-in-action. Both of these concepts are important for nurses and educators because of the practice-based nature of their work. Much of the first section of this chapter dealt with reflection on action (experience) and provided insight into how some of the ways of engaging in this type of retrospective reflection assist learning. In this section of the chapter, we examine three different ways of reflecting-in-action: practical knowledge-in-action, skill acquisition, and praxis.

Tacit Knowing-in-Practice

Schön (1983) contends that another type of reflection—reflection-in-action—is often overlooked completely, and yet is of paramount importance to practitioners. We consider this type of reflection to be important any time that teaching/learning situations require the acquisition of a skill. It is this type of knowing-in-action that Benner and Wrubel (1982) describe in their foundational research that illuminates nursing practice. Schön supports their position and claims that reflection is an intuitive, creative, artistic process, much more than a cognitive/affective process of analysis. Reflection-in-action means that practitioners respond instantaneously to unfamiliar situations in appropriate and skillful ways. As Schön explains:

> When we go about the spontaneous, intuitive performance of actions of everyday life, we show ourselves to be knowledgeable in a special way. Often we cannot say what it is that we know. When we try to describe it, we find ourselves at a loss or we produce explanations that are obviously inappropriate. Our knowing is ordinarily tacit, implicit in our pattern of action and in our feel for the stuff with which we are dealing. It seems right to say that our knowing is in our action. (p. 49)

As with nursing practice, much of teaching practice is chaotic and unpredictable. No matter how much you prepare, you cannot prepare for the unexpected. So much of teaching requires that you to be able to think on your feet, read the situation, and recognize teachable moments. We must be able to think about doing what we are doing while we are doing it.

LEARNING ACTIVITY:
KNOWING AND DOING

Ends in View

In this learning activity, you will explore experiences of knowing-in-action.

Write

In your journal, consider and respond in writing to the following statements and questions.

- Think of a time in your nursing experience when you had to respond to an unexpected situation.
- Describe what happened.
- Who was involved?
- Think about how you knew what to do.
- Try to recall your thinking about the situation. Did you systematically analyze the situation?
- Did you act and then think?

Dialogue

Discuss the situation that you wrote about from your practice with a learning partner. Consider and discuss the following questions: How are your experiences similar or different? How do you account for being able to do something without being able to provide a rationale/analysis for why you did what you did?

Reflect

Contemplate the following question: What is the relationship between knowing and knowing what to do (action)?
Write a full description of this relationship in your journal.

Skill Acquisition: More Than Behavioral Performance

Part of a nurse's education involves learning particular skills. Also, nurses are often called upon to teach particular skills to clients or groups. Usually, people think of skillfulness as being able to do something such as a specific task, for example, being able to give an injection. Benner and Wrubel's (1982) work on nursing practice has contributed significantly to our understanding of this particular type of reflection-in-action in nursing. Their work and that of others (Dreyfus & Dreyfus, 1986) expand our understanding of skillfulness from its usual focus on behavior to include other equally important aspects. There are at least four critical aspects of being skillful.

Perceptual awareness—This aspect refers to the ability to perceive the salient features of a given situation. Certain aspects of a situation stand out as being more important than others.

Behavioral performance—This aspect describes the ability to actually perform a certain task. There is a tendency to focus solely on this aspect of skillfulness.

Discretionary decision making—This refers to the ability to make judgments about what is appropriate as a way to be or what to do in a given situation.

Confidence—This aspect refers to feelings in relation to abilities. Benner and Wrubel did not identify this aspect of skillfulness in their original work. However, our work with learners acquiring skills revealed that confidence is also an important aspect of skillfulness (Hills, 1989).

Benner and Wrubel (1982) also uncovered the critical role of experience in developing skillfulness. Although they claim that there are some aspects of practical knowledge that can only be learned from practice (experience), they also assert that this way of knowing is generally undervalued and not well understood. They explain that western culture traditionally places a premium on abstract reason. As a result, we understand theoretical knowledge better and value it more than knowledge gained through practice or experience (p. 11).

In their research, examining knowledge embedded in nursing practice, Benner and Wrubel (1982) revealed that nurses display different characteristics in their performance depending on their level of development. They identified five levels: novice, advanced beginner, competent, proficient, and expert. What is of interest from

LEARNING ACTIVITY:
SKILL ACQUISITION

Ends in View

This learning activity provides opportunities for you to examine teaching/learning situations that involve skill acquisition.

Write

In your journal, write about a recent experience in which you had to teach someone a skill or you had to learn a skill. Using the four aspects of skillfulness, describe how you paid attention to each aspect.

Dialogue

Share your experiences with your classmates. Discuss the approaches you used to teach this skill. What aspects of skillfulness did you find most difficult to attend to?

a reflection-in-action perspective is the role that experience plays in acquiring skilled knowledge. Benner and Wrubel explain that experience is not mere passage of time or longevity; rather, it is the transformation of preconceived notions and expectations by means of encounters with actual practical situations, that is, reflection-in-action (p. 11). This means that, for situations involving skill acquisition, learners require actual concrete experiences in order to become more proficient or expert practitioners.

Praxis: The Dialect of Reflection and Action

In this section of the chapter, we explore the concepts of reflection and action as a dialectic.

The notion of dialectic is based on the concept of the unity of opposites (thesis; antithesis) and their continual resolution (synthesis) (Webster's Dictionary). The unity of opposites is the recognition of the contradictory, mutually exclusive opposite tendencies in all phenomena and processes of nature (including mind and society).

The condition for the knowledge of all processes of the world in their self-movement, in their spontaneous development, in their real life, is the knowledge of them as a unity of opposites. This conception of the development of knowledge "alone furnishes the key to the self-movement . . . to the transformation into the opposite, to the destruction of the old and the emergence of the new" (Lenin, as cited in Selsam & Martel, 1963, p. 131).

For our emancipatory relational pedagogy, this means understanding the opposing notions of action and reflection and to find synthesis through the process. As Kemmis (1985) explains, reflection is a dialectical process.

> It looks inward at our thoughts and thought processes and outward at the situation in which we find ourselves; when we consider the interaction of the internal and the external, our reflection orients us for further thought and action. Thus, reflection is meta thinking—thinking about thinking in which we consider the relationship between our thoughts and actions in a particular context. (p. 140)

Kemmis argues that reflection is action-oriented, social, and political. We tend to think of reflection as something that happens quietly and personally inside of us. But Kemmis suggests that to do so is "to ignore the very things that give reflection its character and significance: it splits thought from action" (p. 141).

The significance of understanding reflection and action as dialectic is that it frames our understanding in a historical and political context. We do not reflect without reason; we reflect because something has occurred to make us aware of ourselves. We understand that the way we act, to some degree, will impact future events for ourselves and possibly others. From a dialectic position, "reflection is a political act, which either hastens or defers the realization of a more rational, just and fulfilling society" (Kemmis, 1985, p. 140).

So, when people make decisions about their health practices, or learn new ways of being healthy, and by doing so realize that the healthy choices they are making not only improve their health but also the health of the society in which they live, they are engaged in a process of transformational change. These kinds of transformations in perspective are said to have been accomplished through a process of conscientization (Freire, 1972), perspective transformation (Mezirow, 1990), or emancipatory learning (Habermas, 1979). These terms are used to describe situations in which students make fundamental changes in the way that they view themselves, their communities, and their place in the world (Farquharson, 1995).

Mezirow (1990) contends that the most significant learning experiences in adulthood involve critical self-reflection—reassessing the way we have posed problems and reassessing our own orientation to perceiving, knowing, believing, feeling, and acting (p. 13). Perspective transformation is a three-stage process: becoming critically aware of how and why our presuppositions have come to constrain the way we perceive, understand, and feel about our world; reformulating these assumptions to permit a more inclusive, discriminating, permeable, and investigative perspective; and making decisions or otherwise acting upon these new understandings (p. 14). In an emancipatory relational pedagogy, teachers are constantly mindful of potential opportunities to create a situation in which this type of learning can occur. Learning that endures, that is, learning that is retained and easily transferred to other situations, is created through this type of process.

LEARNING ACTIVITY:
Enhancing Society Through Emancipatory Action

Ends in View

In this learning activity, you will consider experiences you have had that are examples of transformative change.

Read

Read the following example of transformative change.

In 1990, I was a very keen jogger and was fairly conscious of what I ate because of my interest in running. One evening, I was talking to someone I had just met—she had recently published a book on vegetarian cooking—and we were discussing the merits of being vegetarian. I had had these types of conversations before and was quite happy with my decision to continue to eat meat. I recall when I was leaving she said light-heartedly, "Remember nothing with a face or a heart!" Later that evening, for some reason I began to view things differently. I became aware of myself acting in habitual ways—I ate meat because that was what I had always done. It was easy. I began to understand that not only did I not need to eat meat but, if I chose not to eat it, I could make a difference to society, to the environment and to thousands of animals that could continue to live! When I awoke the next morning, I decided I would not eat anything with a face or a heart again.

Write

In your journal, write about a time when you had a similar type of transformative experience. Try to recall as many of the details as possible that will assist others in understanding your experience. Write about what it was that heightened your awareness or triggered your reflection. Try to recall your thinking about this situation as you were experiencing it.

Dialogue

Share your experiences with your classmates. Discuss what characteristics your experiences seem to have in common and how they are different. Together, describe the critical aspects that are present in this type of transformative process.

Reflect

In your journal, describe your understanding of this process of transformative change. What aspects seem most important to you? What strategies can you use to encourage this type of transformative change? What are the benefits of engaging in this type of learning?

Freire (1972) considers reflection-in-action as praxis. The constituent elements of praxis are action and reflection, and their relationship is reflexive. Emancipatory action is informed by the dialectal movement from action to reflection and to new action. So, there is a theoretical component, an experience component, and a dialogue component that liberate people to act in ways that enhance society. This dialectal way of viewing reflection-in-action reorients our consideration of this concept from one of searching for understanding or explanation to one of ethical action toward societal good. This is similar to Mezirow's (1990) explanation that conscientization is not merely speculative or theoretical interpretation of an experience, nor is it merely a new way of making sense of nonsensical and oppressive conditions. It is critical reflection—looking back on assumptions underlying our experience and redefining our own being not merely as knowers but as reflective doers (p. 89).

Emancipatory action recognizes the dialectic of action and reflection—it is praxis. Emancipatory action has a different relationship to knowledge than other forms of reflection. From an emancipatory perspective, action flows from practical and theoretical reflection. Grundy (1987) explains that it is action that seeks, through reflective praxis, to make meaning of the social situation in the light of authentic insights into the nature of the socially constructed world (p. 135). If we can understand the world as being socially constructed, we can understand how we can act in the world to change those social constructions toward a more emancipatory position. Emancipatory praxis is realized via the medium of critical self-reflection (Grundy, 1987, p. 188). Viewed from this perspective, "reflection is a power we choose to exercise in the analysis and transformation of the situations in which we find ourselves when we pause to reflect. It expresses our agency as the makers of history as well as the awareness that we have been made by it" (Kemmis, 1985, p. 139).

REFERENCES

Benner, P., & Wrubel, J. (1982). *Skilled clinical knowledge: The value of perceptual awareness. Nurse Educator, 7,* 11–17.

Boud, D., Keogh, R., & Walker, D. (1985). Promoting reflection in learning: A model. In D. Boud, R. Keogh, & D. Walker (Eds.), *Reflection: Turning experience into learning* (pp. 18–40). London: Kogan Page.

Boud, D., Keogh, R., & Walker, D. (Eds.). (1985). *Reflection: Turning experience into learning.* London: Kogan Page.

Boyd, E. M., & Fales, A. W. (1983). Reflective learning: Key to learning from experience. *Journal of Humanistic Psychology, 23*(2), 99–117.

Dreyfus, H. L., & Dreyfus, S. E. (1986). *Mind over machine: The power of human intuition and expertise in the age of the computer.* Oxford, England: Blackwell Press.

Farquharson, A. (1995). *Teaching in practice.* San Francisco: Jossey-Bass.

Freire, P. (1972). *Pedagogy of the oppressed.* New York: Herder & Herder.

Grundy, S. (1987). *Curriculum: Product or praxis?* London: Falmer Press.

Habermas, J. (1979). Communication and the evolution of society. In S. Grundy (Ed.), *Curriculum: Product or praxis?* London: Falmer Press.

Hills, M. (1989). The child and youth care worker as an emerging professional practitioner. *Journal of Child and Youth Care, 4*(1), 17–31.

Kemmis, S. (1985). Action research and the politics of reflection. In D. Boud, R. Keogh, & D. Walker (Eds.), *Reflection: Turning experience into learning* (pp. 139–163). London: Kogan Page.

Lenin, V. I. (1963). Marx's idea of materialism in sociology. In H. Selsam & H. Martel (Eds.), *Dynamics of social change: A reader in Marxist social science* (pp. 82–87). New York: International Publishers.

Mezirow, J. (1990). *Fostering critical reflection in adulthood.* San Francisco: Jossey-Bass.

Murray, J. (1989). Making the connection: Teacher-student interactions and learning experiences. In E. Bevis & J. Watson (Eds.), *Toward a caring curriculum for nursing* (pp. 189–257). New York: National League for Nursing.

Schön, D. A. (1983). *The reflective practitioner: How professionals think.* London: Temple Smith.

Shor, I., & Freire, P. (1987). *A pedagogy for liberation: Dialogues on transforming education.* South Hadley, MA: Bergin & Gavey Publishers.

7
Creating a Culture of Caring

Who am I being that you are not shining?
—Lululemon Athletica Inc., personal communication, 2010

RECENTLY, I HAD THE OPPORTUNITY to attend a management training session that was being facilitated by my daughter who is a culture educator for the western United States for a successful corporate retailer. During this experience, it struck me that this business, which sells athletic clothing, was investing considerable effort and resources into educating its management and staff to create a culture of authenticity within the company. All of their training programs are designed to give them access to what it means to be great in life. As Jenna explains, "The only way to truly be great is to be your true authentic self" (Hills, personal communication, 2010). As I reflected on this notion, I began to wonder about our culture of nursing. Why doesn't nursing proactively teach and nurture its culture of caring?

We believe that nursing, as a discipline and a profession, embraces a culture of caring, yet it is not often articulated nor do nurses deliberate about what it is or how to develop it. As we were developing this idea, it occurred to us that we need to openly recognize the culture aspect that permeates our emancipatory relational pedagogy. By making this culture of caring an explicit component of our pedagogy, we hope to highlight its importance within the education process and to provide nurses with language to express their practice in a way that counters the predominant traditional medically based nursing culture that tends to infiltrate our culture of caring.

In this chapter, we describe creating a culture of caring, the fourth and the final component of our emancipatory relational pedagogy that encapsulates the three others. Just as the embryonic sac surrounds and nurtures a developing embryo, so too does the caring culture surround, nurture, and nourish a student nurse developing within the

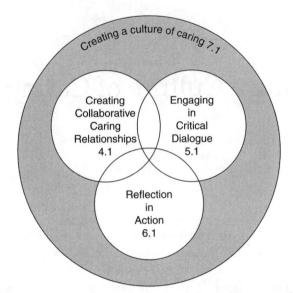

FIGURE 7.1   Interlocking circles of a caring science curriculum.

discipline of nursing. Including this fourth component in our framework highlights the teacher's responsibility to include the component in her/his pedagogical framework (Figure 7.1).

Culture is all the values, perceptions, past associations, past learning, past experiences, and shared mind-sets of all the individuals in a system, many of which are hidden, often unknown, and latent. Our nursing culture includes our taken for granted assumptions, traditions, ways of doing things, and ways of relating to each other. It is sometimes subtle and sometimes not, but it is always there, forming the horizons of our being-in-the-world. We nurses have all experienced this culture in our work places or even when we meet our colleagues in social situations. We have a way of talking, being with each other, relating to one another, and a *shortcut* way of engaging with each other because we share a culture—the culture of nursing. "The culture of nursing has a vital social-scientific role in advancing, sustaining and preserving caring as a way of fulfilling its mission to society and broader humanity" (Watson, 2008, p. 18). If one accepts the proposition that caring is the moral ideal of nursing (Bevis & Watson, 2000; Watson & Ray, 1988), then "teaching caring becomes the moral imperative of nursing educators" (Bevis & Watson, 2000, p. 183).

Nursing is a deeply moral activity requiring the performance of "the most difficult drudgery that human misery generates and some of the most sublime activities that one person ever has the opportunity to do for another" (Bevis & Watson, 2000, p. 183). Nursing is intensely intimate and touches people when they are most vulnerable: often in pain, alone, afraid, and threatened. "If we are to entrust society to nurses hands, teachers must do all that is possible to engender the moral ideal of caring so that caring will compel nurses to act in ways that are positive for these vulnerable individuals and families that are in their trust" (Bevis & Watson, 2000, p. 183). Nurse educators must keep this moral ideal at the forefront of their minds as they plan curricula, develop courses and learning opportunities, and interact with students. The moral ideal of caring, nurses' societal mandate, must infiltrate every moment of everyday that teachers spend with students.

One strategy that assists students to develop a culture of caring is journaling. We have developed a particular strategy for journaling that includes students writing narratives as exemplars from their practice. They are provided with guidelines for developing a story and a framework consisting of domains of nursing practice and relevant quality indicators for critiquing the narrative (Hills, 2002). This process is described more fully in Chapter 14.

For example, one student explained,

> I cannot believe I am in the last three weeks of my first year of nursing . . . it was frustrating at first not doing a lot of hands on work . . . but when it comes down to it . . . the skills have been the easiest of the two to learn. . . . You can *train* almost anyone to do skills but . . . when it comes down to it . . . becoming a part of the patient's health care team, to talk and listen to their needs to understand and believe that patients have rights and beliefs about their own health; that has been the challenge of the first year. . . . I feel that I have gained the confidence and education to successfully achieve what is asked of me as a first year nurse. I have achieved everything from doing a bed bath, to repositioning and turning, to vital signs, medications, enemas, commodes, assisting with feeding understanding the administrative use of oxygen, and charting . . . and the list could go on. . . . Yet, the most important thing that I have learned is that the hands on skills are not the only thing that makes you a nurse . . . it has been exciting to see the pieces fall into place.

As I look back to September, everything seemed to be in its own place: biology, health, professional growth, psychology. Now at the end of my first year as I look back, I realize that it is all becoming one—nursing: I am becoming a nurse!

The following excerpt fully illustrates that if students are taught from an ethic of caring and a moral obligation to act ethically and justly, nothing will stand in their way. This student is attempting to illustrate that nursing is primarily about people and their experiences of health and healing and not about the disease. She explains:

A friend of mine died the other day. I didn't know her very well but in the short time that I knew her I learned a lot about myself. She was in hospital because of a bacterial infection, possibly tuberculosis, and I, as a nursing student, was asked if I wanted to be assigned to care for her. Usually, I am quite eager to get a chance to increase my knowledge about different disease processes and to help others understand their situation, I found myself hesitating to take her as my patient. You see, she was HIV positive. I tried to sort out the different feelings that I was experiencing, the biggest one being fear.

Fear immobilized me. I found that I couldn't think clearly but I was really hoping that I wouldn't have to be her nurse. At that point, I can honestly say that I cared more about myself than I did about her. I worried that somehow getting infected; I thought of what I might be bringing home to my children. I approached her bed with hesitate steps and introduced myself. She was very pleasant and very willing to have a student care for her. She told me that she was also a nurse and that she could remember what it was like being a student. Then, very efficiently, she explained to me about the equipment around her and what the doctors were attempting to do for her while she was in hospital. That day and the next, we spent some time getting to know each other.

Over the next few weeks I chose her as my patient assignment. As my fear dissipated and my knowledge of her illness grew, I began to understand some of what she was going through. I also began to see how other nurses were caught up in their fear. When she would press her call bell, a nurse would answer over the intercom and avoid entering her room. When staff did enter her room, they would put gloves on, even if they were not doing an invasive procedure. No one touched her other than to do something with her equipment, and even then they did not linger long at her bedside. I felt myself bristling at the injustice and unfairness, although I am ashamed to say that I didn't speak up for her when others would make assumptions about her. The world of a student is a double-edged sword. I was only there two days a week and I felt powerless to help her.

As her illness progressed, she experienced behavioral changes and would occasionally lash out at me. Although she was sometimes quite demanding about the way things were done, I was able to look beyond the behavior and appreciate her frustration because others had not taken the opportunity to get to know the person, they saw only the disease and labeled her accordingly.

This woman taught me that fear is natural and that you can get beyond it if we take the first step. When we learn about our fears we are able to look beyond them. I call her my friend because she did everything that friends do for one another, and I tried to do the same for her.

Sadly, though, she died in a hospital filled with people too afraid of illness to care for the person. She had hopes and dreams just as you and I do. Despite the struggle near the end of her life, no one stayed with her to face the inevitable, to calm her fears, to tell her that she would be missed. I wish I had thanked her for helping me to make the journey from ignorance to knowledge. I will miss her, but she will always be with me as will others that have taught me so much about caring. (Hills, 1998, p. 13)

This student is clearly practicing from a moral ethic of caring. Identifying and overcoming her own fear, being cognizant and observing how others were treating the patient, and developing insight into caring practices demonstrate the development of becoming a nurse who will practice from an ethic of caring.

ETHICS OF CARE: A RELATIONAL PERSPECTIVE

The ethics of care is a normative ethical theory; it is a theory about what makes actions right or wrong. It was one of several normative ethical theories that were developed by feminists in the second half of the twentieth century. Carol Gilligan's work in moral psychology (1982) challenged "justice-based" approaches to moral discussion. As she describes, ". . . men tend to embrace an ethic of rights using quasi-legal terminology and impartial principles . . . women tend to affirm an ethic of care that centers on responsiveness in an interconnected network of needs, care, and prevention of harm. Taking care of others is the core notion" (p. 371). Of course, there is nothing preventing men from adopting an ethic of care and we should be careful not to "essentialize" gender differences here, even if the perspective is clearly a feminist one.

Ethics of care contrasts with more well-known ethical views, such as utilitarianism and deontology or Kantian ethics. This sort of outlook is what feminist critics call a "justice view" of morality. A morality of care rests on the understanding of relationships as a response to another in their terms (Gilligan, 1982; Noddings, 2005). So, while the consequentialist and deontological ethical theories emphasize the importance of universal standards and applying them impartially, ethics of care perspectives emphasize the importance of relationships. "The care perspective is especially meaningful for roles such as parent, friend, physician, and nurse, in which contextual response, attentiveness to subtle clues, and the deepening of special relationships are likely to be more momentous morally than impartial treatment" (Beauchamp & Childress, 2001, p. 372). As a result, nurses need to become expert ethicists because they encounter, in a day, more complex moral and ethical dilemmas than most people do in a lifetime. The guidance they need to make decisions when faced with these complex moral issues cannot be found in any rule-bound objective ethical guideline.

> . . . no code of ethics, no list of injunctions, no fear of punishment or hope of reward, and no rules or logic decision tree will effect these tasks of moral education. Only a mentor/ preceptor/teacher modeling a humanistic caring ethic and having a dialogue with students that underscores constructed knowing and encourages them to be personally related to the ethic issues involved can facilitate and enhance students in their moral development for life and for nursing. (Bevis & Watson, 2000, p. 184)

Nurse educators and nurses who work in practice settings where students learn play a critical role in the students' moral development, and they must together nurture this culture of caring if students are to graduate as competent caring nurses. This is not an easy task.

Hegemonic Power

One factor that makes it so difficult to engage in a culture of caring is the existence of hegemonic power. Labonte (1990) describes hegemonic power as

> . . . the ability of a dominant group to control the actions and behaviors of others . . . Hegemonic power is that form of "power-over" that is invisible, internalized and structured within the very nature of our day to day living so that we come to take it for granted. (p. 50)

Hegemonic power is difficult to deal with because it is insidious.
Freire (1972) contends that

> . . . any situation in which A objectively exploits B or hinders his pursuit of self-affirmation as a responsible person, is one of oppression. Such a situation itself constitutes violence, even when sweetened by false generosity, because it interferes with man's ontological and historical vocation to be more fully human. (p. 31)

Freire describes the phenomenon of horizontal violence and suggests that it is a primary characteristic of oppression. It is well documented that this type of oppression and resulting horizontal violence exists in nursing practice. Robinson (1995), for instance, suggests that this is pervasive in our nursing culture. He states: "The extent of our oppression means that we often relate to each other through processes characterized by horizontal violence where we attack each other in response to our subjugated positioning in the culture of health care" (p. 66).

Culture is the sum total of our inter- and inner-subjective life worlds, and it exists below the surface of our outer words, actions, and expressed intentions. This culture is intangible but nevertheless palpable; it has sustaining power that can detour the most elegant and highest ideals. This detouring of vision and dreams and highest ideals is grounded in insecurity, distrust, projection, lack of clear communication, and often fear. Inviting people into a place of caring, of trust, and of meaningful and honest communication can be threatening.

It triggers one's inner relationship with self and other; the inner fears behind the scenes and in the silence of the person's private work that is subtly translated into overt but subtle behaviors. The culture can manifest through an energetic presence of negativity, of critical assessment internally and externally; it becomes threatening because it is facing self, and other through self-disclosure. In the long run, the culture of a faculty, of a subgroup, or of the system will trump all the other aspects of a Caring Science curriculum and all the best efforts toward an emancipatory relational pedagogy. For this reason, it is critical for nurse educators to focus on creating a supportive culture that contrasts with often negative cultural surroundings that nurses experience in their everyday working lives.

One way to overcome this negativity and to live a culture of caring is to choose to be in *power with relationships*. Nurses have a choice about how to use their power. Power can be exerted over those who hold less power: that has been termed *power over*. Power can be exerted against one's peers: that has been termed *horizontal violence*. Where power is shared, either with those in peer positions or with those who have less of it, you are sharing *power with*. Having *power with* relationships is the only power situation wherein a culture of caring can flourish. We could easily make the logical assumption that power is a limited finite resource so that, in order to share power, we must give up some of our limited supply of power. With some forms of power, that might be the case. But, the power that leads us to our humanness is infinite. We have come to know that, the more of this type of power we share, the more we have returned to us.

LEARNING ACTIVITY:

Horizontal Violence

The purpose of this learning activity is to provide opportunities for you to examine the relationship between horizontal violence and teaching/learning.

The following parable was told to us by a former student.

Do you know the story of the crabs and the dolphins?

Did you know that if you put a bunch of crabs in a pot, not a single crab will get out of the pot? They could escape if they were able to climb one on top of the other, but every time one tries, one of the other crabs pulls it down. At times, they even pull each other's legs off!! Not one of the crabs ever escapes!

In contrast, if you watch a school of dolphins, they display a very different type of behavior. When it becomes time to feed, one of the dolphins will swim in the middle and the others will swim around in a circle to protect it. The dolphin in the centre will feed for as long as it wants and when it is finished, the dolphin will swim to the outer circle and another dolphin will swim into the centre and feed for as long as it wants.

So often in nursing, crab behavior is evidenced in the horizontal violence that we display to one another. It is as if we don't know how to behave any differently. So the question then becomes: "Do you want to be a crab or a dolphin?"

Write

In your journal, recall a teaching/learning situation in which you experienced horizontal violence.

Describe what would need to occur to transform these experiences into empowering teaching/learning situations.

Reflect

In your journal, describe how you would promote a *dolphin culture* rather than a *crab culture.*

Another way to overcome such latent underlying energetic cultural drains is to transform; to transmute human fears, apprehensive feelings, and concerns into higher order of love, of compassion and gentleness, of trust, safety, transparency, open and honest communication, and meaningful caring relationships. There must be safe space where nurses are given permission to be human, to be vulnerable, to experience their own healing, and to be accepted and honored with unique gifts as well as frailties. The caring culture has to permeate the consciousness, the intentionality, and the practices of each individual. However, each individual has to be valued and affirmed for her/his contributions, unique reason for being where she/he is, her/his talents, and her/his diverse points of view.

Another successful intervention for cultural transformation is to invite individuals and the collective consciousness of a group into a vision of contributing to something greater than self, to appeal to their role in translating their own human gifts into compassionate human service through their teaching, their roles, whatever they may be: into assisting their colleague, a student, a community group; in offering up their heart and mind to that which inspires and inspirits them for this work that is shared by others and makes a difference; in letting others know they are important and making an important difference; and, in inviting nonconformity, creativity, inspired vision, and ideals beyond the norm.

At the same time the program leader, the head person *holds the space* for self and other to live out this broader and deeper vision of Caring Science, of caring practices, of emancipatory pedagogies. The Caring Science container is large enough to hold the evolving cultural consciousness of the whole, while still sustaining a common vision, a common context, and container for liberation for the evolved consciousness of humanity alike, toward a moral community, a moral culture of caring, and liberation/emancipation.

There has to be room for safe disagreement of individual and group ideas without diminishing of the individuals or the groups. Allowing and creating open space for consensus building, for sharing common human-to-human caring processes and relationships that honor the whole.

Without such elevated vision to appeal to the higher senses of all; without leadership that invites the highest level of ideals and values and ethics into daily practices; without a vision of excellence that affirms the highest ethical caring values of each faculty, each student, each administrator, each employee and holds them in this consciousness, even if the individuals cannot see that for themselves in the moment, then any attempts at creating and sustaining a Caring Science curriculum and emancipatory pedagogies will be undermined and diluted, and ultimately destroy the program by default, not because of the design.

The very same principles for emancipatory pedagogy for faculty-student relations, have to come alive and be lived out at all levels in the program, the curriculum, the classroom, the clinical area, the organizations: between and among faculty to faculty, faculty to student, administrators to administrators, administrators to faculty and students alike. In other words, the caring values and actions, which comprise the entire culture, have to be lived out within the whole; the whole caring consciousness, the liberated thinking and consciousness of emancipation have to be lived out in "caring moments" across the entire organization, from the inside out.

As nurse educators in a Caring Science curriculum, we need to include as part of our emancipatory relational pedagogy a deliberate effort to create a culture of caring in a way that transcends education and becomes a conscious, articulated way of practicing nursing. In order to cultivate this caring way of being, nurse educators must provide precedence for this caring culture over the more traditional bio-medical/technocure culture that has been so dominant in nursing and nursing education. The precedence of this caring culture is the true reflection of the nature of nurse-client and teacher-student relationships, and it is within this context that nurses must be educated if we are to fulfill our mandate to society. As nurse educators who embrace a Caring Science philosophy and theoretical perspective, we are obligated to attend to this development.

Ultimately, the Culture of Caring created by liberated nurse leaders will contribute to our ability to sustain human dignity, to sustain humanity for an evolved human consciousness of connectedness, of unitary views of human-environment, of unity of mindbodyspirit, returning us to the very roots, the very foundation of Caring Science theory, ethics, values, philosophical orientations toward humankind itself.

It is only when we pause, when we are free to critique and find another way to serve our evolved self and others, in safe space, in a communion of caring that we are truly educating for a moral society, a deeply human caring culture that ultimately contributes to world healing and peace.

Finally, with respect to caring culture and open honest communication regarding this book, we too can disclose our motivation, our deepest desire for this book: to offer a transformed vision for Caring Science; to bring forth the ideals and values of Caring Science, to help the evolution of humankind and nursings' ancient and noble contributions to humanity through new ways of understanding education, the liberated human in teaching and learning processes, structure, pedagogies, and informed practices; ultimately to contribute to the evolution of nursing as a discipline and profession that can help sustain human caring and healing for humankind.

REFERENCES

Beauchamp, T., & Childress, J. (2001). *Principles of biomedical ethics*. Oxford, UK: Oxford University Press.

Bevis, E., & Watson, J. (2000). *Toward a caring curriculum. A new pedagogy for nursing*. Sudbury, MA: Jones & Bartlett.

Freire, P. (1972). *Pedagogy of the oppressed*. London: Penguin Books.

Gilligan, C. (1982). *In a different voice*. Cambridge, MA: Harvard University Press.

Hills, M. (1998). Student experiences of nursing health promotion practice in hospital settings. *Nursing Inquiry, 5*(3), 164–173.

Hills, M. (2002). Perspectives on learning and practicing health promotion in hospitals: Nursing students' stories. In L. Young & J. Hayes (Eds.), *Transforming health promotion practice: Concepts, issues and applications* (pp. 229–240). Philadelphia: FA Davis.

Labonte, R. (1990). *Empowerment practices for health professionals*. Toronto, ON: Participation.

Noddings, N. (Ed.). (2005). *Educating citizens for global awareness*. New York: Teachers College Press.

Robinson, A. (1995). Transformative 'cultural shifts' in nursing: Participatory action research and the project of possibility. *Nursing Inquiry, 2*(2), 65–74.

Watson, J. (2008). *Nursing. The philosophy and science of caring* (Rev. Updated ed.). Boulder, CO: University Press of Colorado.

Watson, J., & Ray, M. (Eds.). (1988). *The ethics of care and the ethics of cure: Synthesis in chronicity*. New York: NLN.

III
CREATING A CARING
SCIENCE CURRICULUM

I N THIS UNIT, WE DESCRIBE the phases of the curriculum development process and provide five exemplars of programs and courses
that have used a Caring Science as the philosophy and theory to
develop their curriculum.

There are six chapters in this Unit. Chapter 8 describes the phases
of the curriculum development process within a Caring Science curriculum. A program that was developed based on Caring Science, health
promotion and caring (Collaborative Nursing Program of BC) is used
throughout Chapter 8 to exemplify the developmental processes for a
Caring Science curriculum. The remaining chapters are exemplars from
contributing authors that provide practical examples of ways to develop
and implement a Caring Science Curriculum. Chapter 9 is a contribution
from Boykin, Touhy & Smith that describes a Caring Science Nursing
Program that was developed and implemented over 25 years ago at
Florida Atlantic University. This program continues to be highly successful today. Chapter 10 is a contribution from Lewis, Rogers & Naef
that describes the development of a Human Science curriculum at York
University in Canada. Chapter 11 is a contribution from Hines that describes a doctoral program for advanced nursing practice that was developed at Beth El College of Nursing and Health Sciences at the University
of Colorado, Colorado Springs. Chapter 12 is a contribution from
Rockwood Lane and Samuels that describes courses that were developed based on Caring Science that are currently taught at the College of
Nursing at the University of Florida and at San Francisco State University,
Holistic Studies. The final chapter is a contribution from Sitzman that is
an exemplar of implementing Watson's Theory of Human Caring.

Each of these exemplars is unique, demonstrating different perspectives of a Caring Science Curriculum. Together, they demonstrate
exciting and innovative ways to create a caring curriculum.

8
Curriculum Structure and Design

We have got to get out of our head and into our heart for this next
evolution of humanity
—Barbara Hope, Founding Director WCSI.
(2010 March—Personal Communication)

I N THIS CHAPTER, WE DESCRIBE the processes, structures, and
organizational frameworks, for designing a Caring Science curriculum. In the previous chapters, we have mainly concentrated on
the philosophical underpinnings of a Caring Science Curriculum and
the related transformative relational pedagogy. It is time now to turn
our attention to the structure and design for a Caring Science curriculum. As you know, we can't teach everything all at once, so we need
organizational structures to assist us in this development process. This
is an interesting dilemma because over the past 20 years; largely due to
the "curriculum revolution" of the late 80s and early 90s, we have all
but ignored the structural and design elements of curriculum development. Most of our attention has been focused on the development of
innovative pedagogical approaches. However, we still need to figure
out where to begin and how to proceed in a logical fashion so that our
programs have coherence and some semblance of order.

RECENT CONCEPTUALIZATIONS OF CURRICULUM STRUCTURE AND DESIGN

As discussed in previous chapters dedicated to this topic, emancipatory
relational pedagogical practices, those that are consistent with a Caring
Science curriculum, are a significant factor in implementing a caring
curriculum. Indeed, many, including us, would argue that pedagogy is
the primary influencing factor in curriculum development. That which
actually occurs in the classroom/clinical area among teachers and

students impacts learning the most. However, such components as the development of a program philosophy, the program goals and outcomes, the curriculum design, the way the courses are structured and sequenced, the teacher-student relationship, the learning environment, and the sociopolitical context within which the program is delivered are all significant contributing factors to successful curriculum development. It is not easy to develop a curriculum that captures the complexities of the discipline and that reflects the realities of nursing practice.

Although their focus is not on **caring** science curricula per se, Jillings and O'Flynn-Magee (2007) offer a helpful framework for creating nursing curricula. As they explain,

> the nursing curriculum provides the infrastructure for organizing and delivering content and learning experiences, building cognitive, affective and psychomotor outcomes. The crucial interplay between forms of knowledge, ways of knowing, and the process of curriculum development cannot be understated; if the curriculum is to provide experiences that extend beyond mere content delivery and skill acquisition, it must reflect all dimensions of nursing and in addition, achieve a profound connection with the learner who must ultimately understand and enact the core concepts, theories, and competencies. (p. 384)

Further, they suggest that, currently, we seem to be returning to a more balanced perspective in nursing education where there is focus on the integrity of the curriculum, as well as on teaching/learning processes. They outline six critical phases of curriculum design: contextual elements, philosophy and mission, program outcomes or goals, curriculum framework, curriculum design, and instructional design (p. 395).

Iwasiw Goldenberg, and Andrusyszyn (2009) also focus on the entire curriculum process; however, they pay less attention to pedagogy. They recommend a 12-step process: determining need for change, gain support, organize for curriculum change, plan and implement faculty development, gather data about internal and external contextual factors, agree on philosophical approaches, determine curriculum directions and outcomes, formulate curriculum goals, design the curriculum, design courses, plan evaluation, and plan implementation.

Each of these authors offers valuable and complementary perspectives that are useful in creating a Caring Science curriculum. Both call attention to the contextual factors that can influence curricula development; both promote the importance of the philosophical orientation as being critical to successful implementation; and, both include curricula design, instructional design, and evaluation in their curriculum development process. Iwasiw, Goldenberg and Andrusyszyn add an interesting emphasis on early phases of curriculum development and note some of the particular challenges at the beginning of a curriculum development process. Also, they include, as recommended by Bevis and Watson (1989), a particular focus on faculty development.

CURRICULUM DESIGN AND STRUCTURE FOR DEVELOPING A CARING SCIENCE CURRICULUM

In this section, we incorporate some of these recent conceptualizations of nursing curriculum with processes that are recommended to develop a **caring** curriculum. Even though these processes are described in a linear fashion, curriculum development is actually an iterative process in which each subsequent phase builds on the other while also creating new learning that may result in changing the phase you just completed. It is difficult to describe the recursive nature of the curriculum development process because we can really only describe one thing at a time. However, we will attempt to point out typical places where the iterative process is most apparent. The curriculum processes within a Caring Science curriculum are described in the next section and include the development of the philosophy, program purpose and goals; the curriculum framework that describes the overall organizing framework; the curriculum design that demonstrates the sequencing and structuring courses; the instructional design that includes detailed course development with learning outcomes; a description of teaching methods to be used; and, finally, an evaluation plan that includes strategies for student evaluation, course evaluation, and an overall program evaluation plan.

In this chapter, we define, explain, and give examples of each of these components in order to provide concrete examples of the phases of the curriculum development process. We have used a curriculum that was based in a Caring Science paradigm that was developed collaboratively by five schools of nursing in British Columbia Canada. This program was developed between 1989 and 1992 by a 13-member curriculum development team (Hills, 1998; Hills & Lindsey, 1994; Hills et al., 1994). This program has undergone many iterations and has changed significantly over the years, including adding and changing partners, making many curriculum changes and having many faculty member changes. Our purpose in sharing these experiences is to provide concrete examples of one person's perspective of engaging in the early stages of developing a Caring Science Curriculum.

DEVELOPMENT OF A PHILOSOPHY

Whether you are developing a new program or revising an existing one, developing a philosophical statement is usually where most nurse educators begin. If the curriculum is to claim to be a *Caring Science* curriculum, it obviously needs to incorporate a philosophy that is consistent with Caring Science. We are not suggesting that there is only one theory or one philosophical perspective that is consistent with the Caring Science paradigm; in fact, there are many. The program's philosophical statement basically outlines the faculty members' views, positions, beliefs, and assumptions, and it needs to be alive and evolving. It will guide every other decision you will make, so it is worth spending the time it takes to have it be congruent with all those involved in curriculum development.

This philosophical statement typically consists of a statement about the faculty members' beliefs about nursing, health, and people and their views on teaching and learning—their theoretical and philosophical positions at a minimum. If you are creating a Caring Science curriculum, it should go without saying that a Caring Science philosophy and theory must permeate this philosophical position. At this point, you may want to review Chapter 1 and 2 of this book.

In the Collaborative Nursing Program of British Columbia, several months were spent articulating our philosophy. It is not easy for 13 people with different perspectives to agree on philosophical statements. We engaged in many healthy debates and we developed our "team" capacity by using different team-building exercises. This type of engagement, developing our ability to work as a team, created a sense of coherence with the group, even though we initially held varying perspectives and opinions. For example, we all participated in the Myers Briggs Inventory (© Published by Ross Reinhold & Reinhold Development 1997–2009 for personality preferences). The results and discussions about our personality preferences gave the team members a way to express their discomfort in a situation without feeling "blamed." The example of the philosophical statement below, was one of the iterations that was developed early in our planning process. Reaching this consensus allowed the team to put the philosophy aside for a while so that we could engage in other aspects of the curriculum process.

The Collaborative Nursing Program Philosophy

The philosophy of the collaborative nursing program is informed by humanistic, existential, phenomenological, and socially critical orientations. These orientations are reflected in the way in which the program views persons, health and healing, health care, nursing and curriculum.

PERSONS

Persons refers to human beings, whether they are in an individual, family/group, community, or societal context. They are holistic beings who bring unique meaning to life experiences. People make choices based on the meaning they attribute to their experiences, and their choices are influenced by both internal and external factors. Implicit in the choices people make, is the responsibility to be accountable for the consequences of their actions. Although ultimately alone and self-responsible, people live in relationships with others and are constantly evolving as they interact, and strive toward health.

HEALTH

Health (as described by the World Health Organization) is the extent to which people are able to realize aspirations, satisfy needs, and to change or cope with the environment. The environment comprises all cultural, lifestyle, political-economic, interpersonal, structural, and other ecological factors. Health is a resource, not an object of living: it is a positive concept emphasizing social and personal resources as well as physical capabilities. Promoting health involves enabling people to increase control over and to improve their health (World Health Organization). People in ill health (whether physical, social, psychological, or spiritual) may still consider themselves to be healthy if they are able to lead, what they consider to be, satisfying lives. Health and healing coexist and healing is not simply viewed as the movement along a continuum from illness to health.

HEALTH CARE

The right to health care for all is highly valued by our society and supported by the Canadian nursing profession. Accompanying this right is our belief in equal quality of, and access to, health care through fairly distributed resources within and among our communities. People should be full participants in making decisions about their health.

The complex and changing nature of health care has direct consequences for the way in which nursing is practiced. Nurses have a vital role to play in shaping and responding to the challenges of health care in our society. Nurses must strengthen their mandate and their ability to promote health through continuous professional growth.

NURSING

Nursing is the professionalization of the human capacity to care. Nurses are in a unique position to help people understand their health-related experiences and to embrace their ability to make informed health-care choices. Through caring relationships, nurses inform and involve their clients. This relationship empowers clients to make the best possible choices for their health and enhances the healing process.

Nursing involves a highly complex process of simultaneously using reasoning and intuitive thinking while providing care. Nurses must know, care, manage the context, and deal with the unpredictable; they must assume responsibility for their decisions and their professional growth and be accountable to their profession's standards and ethics.

Nurses work with many other disciplines, and in this multidisciplinary health-care context, nurses provide a unique perspective to client care. The unique role of nursing is the nurse's ability to understand people's situations from their perspective and to participate with them through a caring, informed relationship to promote health responses to life experiences.

CURRICULUM

The curriculum of the Collaborative Program is defined as the interactions that take place between and among students, clients, practitioners, and teachers with the intent that learning take place. Therefore, the quality of the curriculum depends upon the quality of these interactions and students, practitioners, and faculty are equally valued as partners in the learning process. Learning is a reformulation of the meaning of experience and leads to changes in attitudes, feelings, and responses. Learning is critically affected by the learner's concept of self, which is itself learned. The self-concept is enhanced when learners have a need to know, perceive learning as relevant and meaningful, and believe they have a chance of success. It is further enhanced when the learner's past and present experiences are acknowledged, respected, and reflected upon. When learners share the responsibility for identifying learning needs, planning learning experiences, and evaluating programs, their self-confidence increases and they become increasingly self-directed. Learners learn best when they feel cared for and challenged and when they experience success.

Nursing is a discipline that values different ways of knowing. Knowledge is derived from the understanding of self, practice, theory, and research, with each way of knowing informing and influencing the other. This form of praxis is a dialectical process through which knowledge is both derived from and guides nursing practice.

In this philosophy, nursing is seen as "the professionalization of the human capacity to care and nurses are believed to be in a unique position to assist people in understanding their health-related experiences and to encourage them to embrace their ability to make informed health choices" (Hills & Lindsey, 1994, p. 160).

Time Out for Reflection

Go back and review Chapters 1 and 2 of this text.

Consider the beliefs, assumptions, and positions reflected in the philosophy above.

How well does it fit with our current presentation of Caring Science as the disciplinary foundation for nursing.

If you were to write a philosophical statement today, would you find it necessary to refer to other theories such as critical social theory or phenomenology?

Could you write a philosophical statement purely based on Caring Science?

PROGRAM PURPOSE AND GOALS

Once you have reached a place with your philosophical statement that the team feels that they have sufficient consensus to move forward it is time to enter the next phase, developing the program purpose and goals. This is an example of a time when the process can be very iterative. Depending on the team's comfort with moving between two aspects of the curriculum process at the same time, the team can go back and forth between these first two phases, developing the philosophy and the program purpose and goals with relative ease.

The program purpose is a broad public statement that links the philosophy and essential concepts that are embedded in the program to the anticipated outcomes of the program. It describes, in a broad sense, the capacities, abilities, and knowledge of the graduate. The program goals further articulate the program purpose by identifying more

---

Program Purpose

The purpose of this program is to educate nurses to work with individuals, families, groups, or communities from a health promotion perspective and an ethic of caring. The program will provide students with opportunities to develop sensitivity to people's experiences with health and healing. By being cognizant of nurses' professional role, students will learn to work as partners with clients and other health-care providers. Through their understanding and participation in the changing health-care system, graduates will be active participants in creating health for all.

PROGRAM GOALS

The graduate of the program will be able to

- practice nursing with a health promotion caring perspective within a variety of contexts and with diverse client populations;
- be an independent, self-directed, self-motivated, and lifelong learner with a questioning mind and familiarity with inquiry approaches to learning;
- be self-reflective, self-evaluative, accountable, and make clinical judgments based on different ways of knowing, including critical thinking and intuition;
- create and influence the future of nursing practice at a political, social, and professional level by responding to and anticipating the changing needs of society;
- be prepared to meet the professional practice requirements as established by the appropriate legislative body.

specifically how the student will "be" as a graduate. An example of a program purpose and program goals is provided to illustrate these concepts. This example was developed collaboratively by the members of the Collaborative Nursing Program of BC (Hills et al., 1994).

Time Out for Reflection

Consider the following questions and record your responses in your journal.

What relationships exist between the philosophy and the program goals?

Are there concepts included in the philosophy that are not reflected in the program goals? If yes, create a goal to reflect the discrepancy.

Consider the goals for your nursing program? Are they congruent with your philosophy? If not, change one or the other so that they are congruent.

CURRICULUM FRAMEWORK

This phase involves the delineation of core concepts and conceptual maps to guide the learning experience. Over the past several years, nurse educators have been asking, "If nursing education doesn't use a behavioral approach to curriculum design, what should it use?" In many ways, giving up the Tylerian (1949) behavioral approach to curriculum design has created a void in nursing curriculum development and left nursing education struggling to fill that void. A Tylerian approach to curriculum is specific, concrete, and relatively straightforward. You develop your program goals and objectives, decide on terminal objectives for every term, for every course, and then you level the content over the years and semesters being guided by the principle of going from the simple to the complex. This may be an oversimplification, but it illustrates the point that rejecting this structure for curriculum development has provided a space for nurse educators to use their creativity and imagination to create innovative and more nursing-oriented approaches to curriculum development. As Jillings and O'Flynn-Magee (2007) suggests, the nursing concepts that are used to build an organizational framework could come from a nursing model, conceptual framework, nursing theories, or from the mission and outcome statements. "Using these elements as sources of major concepts ensures that the main ideas about nursing roles and competencies and concerns for the recipients of nursing care are included" (p. 395).

The Collaborative Curriculum team in BC used a health promotion framework with an ethic of caring to develop a Caring Science curriculum (Hills, 1998; Hills & Lindsey, 1994; Hills et al., 1994).

The curriculum team in BC used focus groups consisting of nurse educators, nurse administrators, and frontline nurses from hospitals and community, government representatives from the Ministry of Health, the nurses' regulatory organization, and the nurses union to determine what knowledge, attitude, and skills nurses would need to have to practice in the 21st century (Hills et al., curriculum commitment working notes, unpublished working document, 1992). The participants of the focus groups were asked three questions: What will nurses need to know to practice in the 21st century? What will nurses have to be able to do to practice in the 21st century and, what attitudes will nurses require to practice in the 21st century? Similar questions were asked in a study of nurses using a Delphi technique that were not involved in the development of the curriculum, the general nursing population (Beddome et al., 1995).

Data from both experiences were analyzed using a thematic analysis (Van Manen, 2001) and that resulted in the creation of four themes that could be used to organize the nursing content—people's experience with health, people's experience with healing, people's experience with self and others, and people's experience with professional growth; two permeating variables that could be integrated in every semester—caring and health promotion; and, four critical concepts that could be woven into every course—ways of knowing, personal meaning, transitions/time, and context.

Definition of Content Themes

These themes were defined and the definitions were agreed upon by consensus of all members of the curriculum team.

1. *People's experience with health*—defined as the process whereby people realize aspirations, satisfy needs and change and cope with the environment (WHO, 1986).

2. *People's experiences with healing*—defined as the process of becoming increasingly whole, regardless of the medical diagnosis . . . it is the total organismic synergistic response that emerges within the individual and leads to the resolution of the health issue or a peaceful death.

3. *People's experiences with self and others*—defined as the process of understanding the meaning of relationship. Understanding relationships includes self-knowledge and knowledge of others that is achieved through self-reflection, introspection, and interaction. This knowledge of self and others results in the discovery of personal meaning.

4. *People's experiences with professional growth*—defined as the process by which nurses make a difference at a personal, professional, and sociopolitical level.

This framework provided the overall structure to organize the courses within the entire program and is depicted in the diagram below. We used a Celtic knot to represent the interrelatedness of these themes, concepts, and constructs (Figure 8.1).

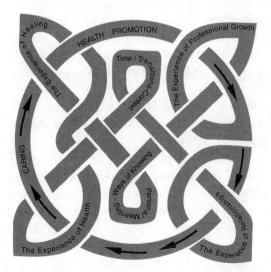

FIGURE 8.1 Framework for collaborative nursing program of BC.

CURRICULUM DESIGN:
STRUCTURING AND SEQUENCING COURSES

Once the framework is in place to provide an overview of the program, courses need to be developed and decisions need to be made about the sequencing of the courses. In addition, electives from other disciplines must be considered and identified. Obviously, you cannot teach everything first and all at once. Several decisions need to be made about what to teach when, what depth of understanding is required at different points in the curriculum, so you need to consider how you will decide what to teach first and what will follow and in what order. This process can be very time-consuming and challenging. Because this process, in some ways more than others, challenges our beliefs about learning, there is often much disagreement among nursing faculty members. This is also the time when decisions need to be made about how the nursing components will interface with the non-nursing aspects of the program, such as electives. For example, some nursing programs believe that students should take liberal arts courses in their first 2 years and do their nursing courses in the senior years of their program. Others believe that nursing courses should occur in every semester beginning with the first and be integrated throughout the curriculum. No matter what the decision, the program philosophy of caring must be visible in the decisions that are made.

In the development of Collaborative Nursing Program of BC, all nursing content was organized under the four themes identified above and these themes were sequenced and structured throughout the 4 years of the program. Initially, a matrix was created simply to place the different courses leveled throughout the curriculum into different semesters. For example, Health 1 was placed in semester 1, Health 2 in semester 2, Health 3 in semester 3, etc. Each of the four themes was placed in the matrix in this way.

Each course within a theme was then further developed by a predetermined focus. For example, the theme people's experience with health and healing occurred in each semester but had a different focus and level of complexity, semester to semester. In year 1, semester 1, the course on people's experiences of health and healing focused on *health* and what it means to be healthy. Students learn about health by examining their own health and that of others and by hearing people's perceptions of health. In year 1, semester 2, the course on people's experiences of health and healing focused on people living with chronic diseases. The people and health focus is maintained but students learn particularly about people's experiences of living with a chronic disease such as diabetes, asthma, etc. In Year 2, semester 3, the course on people's experiences with health and healing focuses on people's experiences of living with episodic health challenges, and in semester 4, they learn about people's experiences of living with acute episodic health challenges.

All themes of nursing content were distributed throughout the curriculum in a similar way (Figure 8.2).

There are at least two important points about the structure and sequencing of these courses. The nursing faculty was committed to creating courses that truly reflected nursing, and it accomplished that by using language, concepts, and knowledge that are within nursing's domain of practice, not medicine's. This was a struggle because for at least 40 years we had been designing nursing curricula based on medicine's disease treatment-cure model. Second, the nursing faculty wanted all courses to reflect its commitment to its philosophy and program goals. Again, it accomplished this by keeping a health promotion perspective and an ethic of caring at the forefront in all course development.

INSTRUCTIONAL DESIGN: COURSE DEVELOPMENT AND LEARNING OUTCOMES

This phase focuses on detailed course development including explicating which courses will be developed by whom, what content will be taught, what learning outcomes will be anticipated, and what teaching and evaluation strategies will be used. Also, it involves articulating how each course will support the program purpose and goals and how philosophical integrity will be achieved and maintained.

Each course usually has a course title, a course description, and a purpose. These essential elements are typically published in an institutional calendar or catalogue. Additional course materials are usually developed for students that include teaching strategies, expectations of students and teachers, and methods of evaluation. In a Caring Science curriculum, courses need to be designed to maximize student engagement, promote caring teaching student relations, and have evaluation strategies that are emancipatory and caring.

	SEPTEMBER - DECEMBER		JANUARY - APRIL		MAY - AUGUST	
YR.I	**SEMESTER 1**		**SEMESTER 2**			
	HEALTH I (N)	(0-0-3-1)	HEALTH II (N)	(0-0-3-0)	PRACTICUM	(0-20-4-0)
	PRO.GROWTH I (N)	(0-4-4-0)	S & O II	(3-0-0-0)	7 WEEKS	
	HEALTH SCIENCE I	(3-0-0-3)	ELECTIVE	(3-0-0-0)		
	S & O I (PSYCHI)	(3-0-0-0)	HEALTH SCIENCE II	(3-0-0-3)		
	PACKAGE I • •	(3-0-0-0)	NURSING PRACTICE I (N)	(0-8-2-3)		
	TOTAL HOURS	(24)	TOTAL HOURS	(28)	TOTAL HOURS	(24)
YR.II	**SEMESTER 3**		**SEMESTER 4**			
	HEALING W.S.I (N)	(0-0-0-6)	PROF.GROWTH II (N)	(0-0-3-0)	W.E. I (CO-OP)	
	NURSING PRACTICE II (N)	(0-12-4-0)	HEALING W.S.II (N)	(0-0-3-6)		
	HEALTH SCIENCE III	(3-0-0-0)	NURSING PRACTICE III (N)	(0-12-4-0)		
	PACKAGE II	(3-0-0-0)	HEALTH SCIENCE IV	(3-0-0-0)		
	TOTAL HOURS	(24)	TOTAL HOURS	(28)		
YR.III	**SEMESTER 5**		**BRIDGE**		**SEMESTER 6**	
	PROF.GROWTH III (N)	(0-0-3-0)	BRIDGE IN		HEALTH IV (N)	(0-0-3-0)
	PHILOSOPHY	(3-0-0-0)	HEALTH (N)	(0-0-3-0)	S & O III (N)	(0-0-3-0)
	HEALTH III (N)	(0-0-3-0)	PRO.GROWTH (N)	(3-0-0-0)	HEALTH SCIENCE V (N)	(3-0-0-0)
	NURSING PRACTICE IV (N)	(0-12-4-0)	HEALTH SCIENCE (N)	(3-0-0-0)	STATISTICS	(3-0-0-0)
	PROF.GROWTH IV	(3-0-0-0)	NURSING PRACTICE (N)	(0-8-3-0)	NURSING PRACTICE V (N)	(0-6-3-0)
			PACKAGE	(3-0-0-0)		
	TOTAL HOURS	(28)	TOTAL HOURS	(21)	TOTAL HOURS	(21)
			BRIDGE OUT			
			HEALING (3 WK.) (N)	(0-0-4-8)		
			PRECEPTORSHIP			
			(37.5 HRS. X 11 WK.) (N)			
			CONTINUING STUDENTS			
			W.E. II (CO-OP)			
YR.IV	W.E.III		**SEMESTER 7**		W.E.IV	
			PROF GROWTH V (N)	(0-0-3-0)		
			PROF GROWTH VI (N)	(0-0-3-0)		
			PACKAGE III	(3-0-0-0)		
			S & O IV	(3-0-0-0)		
			NURSING PRACTICE VI (N)	(0-6-3-0)		
			TOTAL HOURS	(21)		
YR.V	**SEMESTER 8**					
	INDEPENDENT					
	CLINICAL STUDIES	21 HR. WK. x 13 WKS. (N)				
	RATIO 1:20					

Before the Bridge
Seminar 1:32
Clinical 1:08
Lab 1:10

After the Bridge
Seminar 1:32
Clinical 1:16

Preceptorship 1:20

• • PACKAGE = CHOICE BETWEEN SOCIOLOGY, ANTHROPOLOGY, PSYCHOLOGY, PHILOSOPHY

(0-0-0-0) = 1 ST # REFLECTS CLASS ROOM: 2ND # REFLECTS CLINICAL: 3 RD # REFLECTS SEMINAR: 4TH # REFLECTS LAB

FIGURE 8.2 Course content by theme—CNPBC.

Course design and development is another of those processes in curriculum development that is iterative. Courses inevitably change over time as faculty members receive feedback from students and revise the course. This keeps the curriculum alive and evolving.

In the Collaborative Nursing Program of BC, themes teams were constituted to develop each of the courses. Course content had already been articulated within each of the nursing content themes (Figure 8.3) so the work now concentrated on sorting content over semesters and years of the curriculum.

Because this program was developed across five different nursing programs within five different institutions, the curriculum team worried about program integrity throughout the curriculum development process. One way that this was handled was for the team to focus on the nursing concepts to be taught and to develop learning activities (discussed below) that would encourage the learning of those concepts. As a result, the team developed a "virtual extensive library" of learning activities for each course. A faculty member who was assigned to teach that course had multiple learning activities to choose from, but they all were focused on learning the content, competencies, and skills for that course.

Exemplary curriculum based on health promotion

	Semester 1	Semester 2	Semester 3
Year 1	Health	Chronic Health Challenges	Practicum
Year 2	Episodic Health Challenges	Complex Episodic Health Challenges	Perceptorship/ Co-op Work
Year 3	Prevention	Perceptorship	Health Promotion
Year 4	Perceptorship/ Co-op Work	Societal Health	Perceptorship/ Co-op Work Experience
Year 5	Individual Area of Focus		

FIGURE 8.3 Content themes by semester.

TEACHING METHODS

This phase has been covered quite extensively in Chapters 3, 4, 5, 6, and 7, so there are only a couple of additional concepts that we need to add at this point. One of the most useful strategies for teachers who want to create a Caring Science curriculum and use emancipatory relational pedagogy is to learn how to develop learning activities. As Bevis states, "It is not what the teacher says or does that is important; it is what the teacher has the students do that is important in the overall scheme of education" (Bevis & Watson, 1989, p. 125).

Bevis and Watson, 1989 recommend that teachers become meta strategists; using teaching methods of engagement. We spend considerable time thinking about how to design teaching/learning experiences that will create the dance between theory and practice. We strategize about the types of questions to ask that will provoke critical reflection in ourselves and our students. Although it is important to have knowledge of the content area, we usually spend more time thinking about what I don't know about the topic or issue than about what we do know. We try to think about how we view an issue and why that is the case. We try to determine what questions we need to ask to better understand the relationship between the elements of the issue at hand. We become curious about why others think differently or the same as we do about an issue.

But, how do we give order to these questions so we know how to progress? You have already learned some strategies for doing this, such as Wallerstein and Bernstein's SHOWED method. Another way to structure teaching/learning experiences is by using learning activities (Bevis & Watson, 1989). As you have experienced throughout this book, we use learning activities to structure teaching/learning encounters.

CREATING LEARNING ACTIVITIES

Engaging in critical dialogue requires considerable planning and thoughtfulness. We use learning activities to *structure* dialogue in a teaching/learning situation. Learning activities (Bevis & Watson, 1989) as they are used here have particular meaning and structure and consist of several component parts.

The following guidelines for developing learning activities were developed by Bevis and Hills to be used specifically in the development of the Collaborative Nursing Program of BC.

Guidelines and Structure for Developing Learning Activities

Overview

- Use a "hook" to grab the learner's interest
- Describe why this learning activity should be chosen
- Answer the question "So what?"
- Describe how this learning activity is connected to other learning activities

Ends in View

- Outline the purpose of the learning activity
- Describe the opportunities for learning it will provide

In Preparation

- Provide structure—this may be in the form of questions or readings
- May ask student to reflect on previous experience

In Clinical or Real World

- Provide experiential-based activity
- Give clear instructions
- Relate activity to overview

In Seminar

- Provide structure to analyze information
- Consider how analysis will address
  - critical thinking
  - caring connection

- praxis
- ways of knowing
- Pose questions to help learner derive meaning
- Remember that the purpose of analysis/synthesis is to
  - increase learner's ability to recognize patterns
  - increase learner's ability to increase generalizability
- Remember to include an elastic clause for student input:
  - How would you (the learner) like to change the learning activity?
  - What would you like to do instead that is comparable?

Write

Have students keep a journal throughout the course. Having opportunities to write encourages critical thinking and reflection.

Dialogue

- Encouraging students to have at least a learning partner or a study group is even more preferable. Discussing their ideas, writings, and experiences assists students to become knowledgeable about issues, confident in their own thinking, and reflective about their practice.
- With your learning partners or study group, discuss your experiences of having completed the learning activities for this course. Consider if there are other ways that you might structure a teaching/learning experience.

Reflect

- Adding a reflection component to the learning activity assists students to become reflection practitioners and to develop insight into their learning and practice.
- This structure of learning activities has proven to be particularly helpful in the development of our collaborative curriculum; it provided faculty members with a way of maintaining some consistency

in pedagogical practices across numerous sites and in the development of our courses for off-campus delivery.

CRITERIA FOR CRITIQUING LEARNING ACTIVITIES

The following criteria were developed by Bevis and Hills to be used to critique learning activities that were developed for the Collaborative Nursing Program of BC.

- The theoretical base is explicit—learning activities are scholarly.
- There are clearly labeled headings.
- The learning activity is directive—learners are provided with clear directions.
- The learning activity contains only one learning activity.
- Learning activities that belong together are arranged in clusters.
- There is an elastic clause—to provide flexibility for the learner.
- The learning activity is reality based.
- The learning activity addresses critical aspects of the curriculum, program, or course.
- There is a similar format for the learning activities so that learners can anticipate what follows.

EVALUATION PLAN

The final phase of the curriculum development process is the design of an evaluation plan. This plan should include strategies for evaluating individual courses and an overall strategy for evaluating the program. In addition, strategies for evaluating student classroom and clinical performance need to be developed as part of the plan. Although it is beyond the scope of this book to describe program evaluation (there are many excellent books written on the subject), we have included concepts of evaluation related to assessing student performance in Unit 4. However, it is important to note that the planning for evaluation occurs simultaneously with curriculum development and is integral to the development process.

In addition to the evaluation plan that faculty members and schools of nursing are interested in for their own purposes, nursing programs are regulated and are required to meet Standards of Practice guidelines designated by their governing bodies. An evaluation plan for this type of external evaluation must also be planned.

REFERENCES

Beddome, G., Budgen, C., Hills, M. D., Lindsey, A. E., Duval, P. M., & Szalay, L. (1995). Education and practice collaboration: A strategy for curriculum development. *The Journal of Nursing Education, 34*(1), 11–15.

Bevis, E., & Watson, J. (Eds.). (1989). *Toward a caring curriculum: A new pedagogy for nursing*. New York: National League for Nursing.

Hills, M. (1998). Student experiences of nursing health promotion practice in hospital settings. *Nursing Inquiry, 5,* 164–173.

Hills, M., & Lindsey, E. (1994). Health promotion: A viable curriculum framework for nursing education. *Nursing Outlook, 42*(4), 158–162.

Hills, M., & Lindsey, E., Chisamore, M., Basset-Smith, J., Abbott, K., & Fournier-Chalmers, J. (1994). University-college collaboration: Rethinking curriculum development in nursing education. *The Journal of Nursing Education, 33*(5), 220–225.

Iwasiw, C. L., Goldenberg, D., & Andrusyszyn, M. A. (2009). *Curriculum development in nursing education*. London: Jones Bartlett.

Jillings, C., & O'Flynn-Magee, K. (2007). Knowledge and knowing made manifest: Curriculum process in student-centered learning. In L. Young & B. Paterson (Eds.), *Teaching nursing: Developing a student centered learning environment*. Philadelphia: Lippincott, Williams, & Wilkins.

Tyler, R. (1949). *Basic principles of curriculum and instruction*. Chicago: The University of Chicago Press.

Van Manen, M. (2001). *Researching lived experience*. University of Western Ontario, Althouse Press.

World Health Organization. (1986). *Ottawa charter*. Geneva, Switzerland: Author.

Young, L., & Paterson, B. (2007). *Teaching nursing: Developing a student-centered learning environment*. Philadelphia: Lippincott, Williams & Wilkins.

9

Evolution of a Caring-Based College of Nursing

Anne Boykin, PhD, RN
Theris A. Touhy, DNP, CNS
Marlaine C. Smith, RN, PhD, AHN-BC, FAAN

HISTORY AND BACKGROUND OF THE PROGRAM

THE STORY OF THE EVOLUTION of the nursing program in the Christine E. Lynn College of Nursing at Florida Atlantic University (FAU) was originally described in a book written by the faculty and edited by the dean: *Living a Caring-Based Program* (Boykin, 1994). Following is a description of the early years of the program as presented in Chapter 1 of this book. Our evolution is a story of commitment, passion, innovation, and caring for an idea of nursing and helping it grow. The program began in 1979 with the establishment of an upper-division nursing program for registered nurses, the first such program at a public university in our area. Although our numbers were small (4 faculty members, a consultant Director, and 10 RN to BSN students), we were blessed with an opportunity that allowed us the freedom to create our concept of nursing and to explore innovative teaching strategies. We were not yet aware of the many implications of our task, nor were we bound by what had come before.

Our talented RN to BSN students were leaders in the nursing community and masters of their skill. They had achieved a high level of success in the profession, and they challenged us with the question: "We are expert nurses, what more do we need to learn about nursing?" They forced us to continually think about nursing as a concept, apart from skills, techniques, and the medical model in which we had all been schooled. We shared our ideas about what was important in nursing practice and our hopes and dreams for how nursing practice could be improved. As we studied the concept of nursing and its essence, we began to filter nursing from nonnursing content in an effort to articulate the essence of our discipline. Among our early influences were the values and teaching work of Sid Simon and Jay Clark (1975) and Diane Ustal's (1977) work on values clarification in nursing. Our teaching-learning philosophy was one of openness and mutuality, which yielded a healthy respect for learning from and with each other. The theories of Martha Rogers (1970), Madeline Leininger (1981), Jean Watson (1979), and Paterson and Zderad (1976) assisted us to more fully reflect on the discipline of nursing. Caring for self and other emerged as an essential framework for nursing in those early years.

With plans to begin a generic program in 1982, additional faculty members were hired and a full-time Director was appointed. The dialogue on caring as a concept of great depth in the discipline took on new dimensions. Our original curriculum, like many others at that time, was organized using a general systems theory framework. Yet, our philosophy at that time hinted at our real values, as illustrated in this statement from the 1981 philosophy: "The foundation of professional caring is the blending of humanistic, scientific, and nursing theories. Humanistic caring is the creative, intuitive, and cognitive aspects of the helping process." Through the process of preparing for accreditation, faculty members began to identify those aspects of the philosophy, and particularly the framework for the curriculum, which did not fully express where we were in our thinking about nursing.

This was an exciting time for faculty members to focus on the essence of the discipline, our beliefs about nursing, and how we could create a program of study that reflected these beliefs and values. Faculty members began to ask difficult questions, such as: Do we want to continue teaching nursing as we have been, or shall we take the risk and ask the question "what is the content of the discipline that should be taught?" All faculty members realized that the classroom content being taught was predominantly medical science. We struggled to know what, in fact, was the content of the discipline. The process of discovery began by evaluating the syllabi for existing courses. The first step was easy. All the content that was not specific to nursing was sorted out. A decision was made to place all of the pathophysiology, pharmacology, and assessment content into separate courses. The question became, what content would fill the remaining gaps? If we were no longer approaching the study of nursing through diseases, then what was the content of the discipline to be studied?

We began to meet regularly, and by sharing our individual stories of nursing practice, we began to believe that if they were shared with students, the content of nursing would be known. This process was long, confusing, exciting, scary, and continuous. Omission of its details should not lead the reader to believe the process was simple and without painful struggles. Throughout our dialogue, the importance of caring as a unique concept in nursing continued to unfold. Many factors nurtured and influenced the growth of this concept. Mayeroff's book, *On Caring* (1971), was and continues to be a required text in our program because it offers a generic way of knowing self and other as caring person. Paterson and Zderad's book, *Humanistic Nursing* (1976), also had a significant influence on the evolution of the curriculum. Their ideas about the phenomenon of nursing, nursing situations, and call and response seemed to fit with our concept of nursing. Carper's (1978) ways of knowing helped broaden our understanding of the range of knowledge needed to study and practice nursing. We questioned: what it means to be caring; how caring is lived in nursing; can caring be taught; and how best to teach caring? Roach's exquisite works describing the manifestations of caring and the attributes or qualities demonstrated in the professionalization of caring helped us answer these questions and move forward to establish a program of study grounded in caring. The works of many other scholars were brought forward for ongoing dialogue. The theory of Nursing as Caring (Boykin & Schoenhofer, 2001) has had a significant influence on our philosophy and programs of study. However, our faculty did not ascribe to any particular framework; instead, we created our own statements of belief on caring.

Many things have changed in the 31 years since we began caring for an idea of nursing and helping it grow (Figure 9.1). We now have 45 faculty members and 1,300 students in programs of study at the baccalaureate, masters, and doctoral (DNP and PhD) levels. What has not changed is our passion for nursing, the love of nursing as a unifying body, and the belief that nursing offers a unique and invaluable service to human persons—caring. Through the scholarly work of

Florida Atlantic University
Christine E. Lynn College of Nursing

STATEMENT OF PHILOSOPHY

Nursing is a discipline of knowledge and a field of professional practice grounded in caring. Scholarship and practice in nursing require creative integration of multiple ways of knowing. Nursing makes a unique contribution because of its special focus: nurturing the wholeness of persons and environment through caring. Caring in nursing is a mutual human process in which the nurse artistically responds with authentic presence to calls from person(s). The experience of nursing takes place in nursing situations: lived experiences in which the caring between the nurse and person(s) fosters well-being within a co-creative experience. Nurses participate with members of other disciplines to advance human understanding to enhance personal and societal living within a global environment.

Person is viewed as a unique individual dynamically interconnected with others and the environment in caring relationships. The nature of being human is to be caring. Humans choose values, culturally derived, which give meaning to living and enhance well-being. Well-being is creating and living the meaning of life. The well-being and wholeness of persons, families, groups, communities and societies are nurtured through caring relationships.

Beliefs about learning and environments which foster learning are derived from an understanding of person, the nature of nursing and nursing knowledge, and the mission of the University. Learning involves the creation of understanding through the integration of knowledge within a context of value and meaning. A supportive environment for learning is a caring environment. A caring environment is one in which all aspects of the human person are respected, nurtured, and celebrated. The learning environment emphasizes collegial relationships with faculty and students.

The above fundamental beliefs concerning Person, Nursing, and Learning express our values and guide the endeavors of the Faculty. Faculty of the College of Nursing believe in the values and goals of higher learning and support the Florida Atlantic University mission of education, scholarship and service.

Revised 8/05, Christine E. Lynn College of Nursing philosophy.

FIGURE 9.1 Philosophy of the Christine E. Lynn College of Nursing.

our faculty members and our students, we continue to reflect upon, develop, celebrate, and share the values that called each of us to the human service of nursing. We continue to evolve in our understanding of teaching nursing grounded in caring and extending and developing the study of the concept of caring. It is our belief that without a focus on caring as an essential domain of nursing knowledge, the nature of nursing cannot be fully understood. Our commitment to creating a College founded on caring includes not only the study of nursing but the cocreation of an environment to foster knowing of each other as caring persons and the gifts we bring to this process.

CREATING A CULTURE OF CARING

Beliefs and values of the faculty not only guide the design, implementation, and evaluation of a caring-based program but they also frame a way of being in relationship with self and other. The Dance of Caring Persons (Boykin & Schoenhofer, 2001) is the model used to express caring relationships. This model (Figure 9.2), etched in the terrazzo floor of the lobby of the College of Nursing building, serves as a constant reminder of right ways of relating grounded in respect for and valuing of each person. The flat aspect of a circle conveys that each dancer brings unique gifts to the work of the College. No one person's

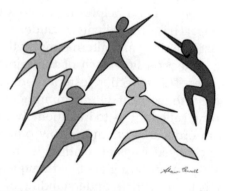

FIGURE 9.2 The dance of caring persons.

gifts are more important than another's—just different due to role. In this way, the College's structure is not represented in a traditional organization chart, but a circular, flat structure depicting interrelationships rather than hierarchy (see Models of Relating at http://nursing .fau.edu/index.php?main=4&nav=578). Each person is viewed as special and caring. Each role is essential to accomplishing the mission and goals of the College. The circle is open as there is always room for others to join the dance. The intent of all dancers is to know other as caring person and support each other in living caring uniquely. The ongoing challenge is to be open to knowing caring in the moment. One aspect of the dance is that each person is engaged in the lifelong process of growing in knowing self and other as caring person.

An explicit understanding of what it means to be a person provides direction for being in all relationships—personal and professional. Select excerpts from the College philosophy that guide the continual unfolding of a culture grounded in caring include:

- Person is viewed as a unique individual dynamically interconnected with others and the environment in caring relationships.
- The nature of being human is to be caring.
- A caring environment is one in which all aspects of human person are respected, nurtured, and celebrated.

These beliefs are intended to directly guide our way of being. The declaration that all persons are caring and engaged in caring relationships calls for an understanding of what it means to live caring both in the ordinariness of life and uniquely in the practice of nursing. Mayeroff's (1971) caring ingredients offer a helpful framework for knowing self and other as caring. These ingredients include: knowing, honesty, courage, hope, trust, humility, and alternating rhythm. Faculty members and students reflect on how each of these ingredients is lived uniquely in their lives. This reflection fosters an understanding of self living caring moment to moment. Our commitment to the belief that all persons are caring called for us to intentionally come to know self as caring person in order that we may know others as caring. This personal knowing changed ways of relating. It brought forth the realization that expressions of caring are lived uniquely by each person and the challenge is to grow in an understanding of what it means to live caring.

Examples of strategies as a faculty to facilitate knowing of self as caring include:

- Retreats that focus time on centering self in order that one may have heightened awareness of the unique ways of living caring;
- Structured time for informal dialogue with colleagues on what it means to be a faculty member in a caring-based program;
- Designated time for meditation;
- Opportunities to experience various ways of caring for self, that is, through yoga classes or participating in therapeutic touch sessions offered at the College;
- The study of nursing with students focused on knowing self and other as caring person.

Opportunities for students to know self as caring are integrated throughout their program of study. Students are first introduced to the concept of caring as they tour the College. The building itself was designed to be a "teacher" of caring. When we received the remarkable ten million dollar gift from Christine E. Lynn (matched by the State of Florida), we decided that our new home would be an expression of caring. It is a healthy, healing place built on principles of sustainability and a commitment to transform nursing education through creation of healing spaces. It is a structure that celebrates and honors the traditions of nursing. Many spaces were intentionally designed to support reflection and knowing of self as caring person. These spaces include a sacred space for meditation, several "outdoor" rooms embraced by a garden with a labyrinth, and a holistic practice area. Students systematically focus on knowing self as caring. In the course, Caring for Self, students are engaged in exploring knowing self as caring person and in examining the literature on caring for self.

Each student is their own "laboratory," experiencing and learning how to make choices supportive of personal well-being. Examples of activities from various courses that support knowing self include the following:

- Weekly nursing practice logs where students are invited to reflect on knowing and encountering self and other as they contemplate "Who are the nurse and nursed as caring persons?"; "How are the nurse and nursed expressing caring in the moment?"; and "How did the nurse and nursed grow through caring?"

- Intentional experiential strategies are integral to many courses. In the course, Nursing Situations: Caring for Self, Others and the Environment, students use Mayeroff's (1971) caring ingredients as a way to know self as caring. They ask, "How do I live my knowing, trust, hope, alternating rhythm, courage, humility and patience in the ordinariness of life?" Cameron's book, *The Artist's Way* (1992), guides experiential activities and coming to know self and other as the creator of one's life. The course concludes with the eight principles that Eknath Easwaran (1989) described in *The Compassionate Universe: The Power of the Individual to Heal the Environment.*

THE SHARED STUDY OF NURSING

The shared study of nursing (commonly called the curriculum) is derived from our philosophy and is based on the understanding of nursing as a professional discipline grounded in caring. The unique focus and defining characteristic of nursing as a social and human service is nurturing the wholeness of persons and environment through caring (Christine E. Lynn College of Nursing, 2005). Caring is the essential value held dear to those who choose to be members of a helping profession. To study nursing is to study caring, to grow in understanding of self and other as caring person, and to be committed to the development of caring knowledge and the value of caring to the health and wholeness of persons nursed (Boykin & Schoenhofer, 2001; Touhy & Boykin, 2008).

From the fundamental beliefs of the faculty, five major themes guide all course objectives in the programs and provide a mode of inquiry for each course:

- Images of nurse and nursing
- Nursing as a discipline of knowledge
- Nursing as a profession
- Wholeness of persons connected with others and the environment through caring
- Nursing as the nurturing of wholeness of others through caring

Table 9.1 provides course descriptions and sample objectives for the curricular theme, nursing as a discipline of knowledge for the foundational courses in undergraduate and graduate programs. The

TABLE 9.1 Curricular Theme: Nursing as a Discipline of Knowledge

NUR 3115: Introduction to Nursing as a Discipline and Profession (UG)

Course Description: An introduction to nursing as a distinct discipline of knowledge and a unique professional service. Foundational concepts studied include: Images of nurse and nursing, nursing as a discipline of knowledge, nursing as a profession, nurturing the well-being and wholeness of persons connected with the environment, and the practice of nursing.

Course Objectives: Express an understanding of nursing as a discipline of knowledge, including:

a. differentiating among characteristics of disciplines of knowledge

b. expressing ways of knowing fundamental to nursing

c. discerning major theoretical conceptions of nursing

d. appreciating the conception of nursing held by FAU College of Nursing faculty

e. describing modes of inquiry

NGR 6110: Advanced Nursing Practice Grounded in Caring (Masters)

Course Description: A detailed examination of caring as an essential concept for nursing practice, research, administration, and education. Major contributions to an understanding of caring from the humanities, sciences and nursing (including transcultural nursing) are surveyed. Emphasis will be given to conceptualizations of caring in nursing and philosophical literature. The student will examine the implications of caring in nursing using multiple ways/patterns of knowing.

Sample Course Objective: Advance the discipline of nursing through practice and research

a. Synthesize advanced knowledge of caring in nursing as a dynamic, relational, cocreative, transactional and transcultural process that facilitates choice-making of clients and significant others for well-being, health and healing in health care and nursing situations.

NGR 7116: Caring: An Essential Domain of Nursing Knowledge (Doctoral)

Course Description: Advanced study of caring as an essential domain of nursing knowledge grounding nursing practice, research, administration and education. Caring in nursing is studied from ontological/existential, epistemological, ontical, metaphysical, theoretical, historical, sociocultural and other perspectives.

1. Sample Course Objective: Advance the discipline of nursing through practice and research by:

   a. Analyzing how caring has been studied and researched and how caring should be studied.

   b. Evaluating the evolution of ideas about caring as expressed in caring theory, practice and research.

   c. Critiquing existing theories of caring as guides for nursing practice and research.

   d. Identifying gaps in knowledge that inform the development of a research focus.

foundational undergraduate course is *Introduction to Nursing as a Discipline and Profession*; master's level course is *Advanced Nursing Practice Grounded in Caring*; and doctoral course, *Caring: An Essential Domain of Nursing Knowledge.*

NURSING SITUATIONS: THE CONTEXT FOR KNOWING NURSING

The concept of the nursing situation guides the study of nursing for faculty members and students in all nursing courses. Faculty members believe that the experience of nursing takes place in nursing situations: lived experiences in which the caring between the nurse and client fosters well-being within a cocreative experience (Christine E. Lynn College of Nursing, 2005). The nurse enters the world of the person nursed with the intention of knowing the other as caring person and coming to know how the other is living caring in the situation and expressing hopes for growing in caring. Within the nursing situation, the nurse attends to calls for caring and creates caring responses that nurture personhood (Boykin & Schoenhofer, 2001).

In each nursing situation there are calls for nursing and a response from the nurse. Identification of the calls for nursing arises from the nurses' intentional full engagement with the one nursed and from the ability of the nurse to draw on a broad knowledge base in order to understand the particular situation. Through authentic presence, as caring person, the nurse is able to enter the world of the other, come to know the other, hear calls for nursing, and respond appropriately to nurture wholeness. Inquiry into nursing situations facilitates student understanding of nursing as a discipline and a professional practice grounded in caring.

In the study of nursing situations, there are no "standard" calls or responses—no predetermined goals or plan of care based on a medical diagnosis. The person nursed is always the focus of the nursing situation. Boykin and Schoenhofer (2001) reflected:

> The challenge for nursing is not to discover what is missing, weakened, or needed in another but to come to know the other as caring person and to nurture the person in situation specific, creative ways. We no longer understand nursing as a "process" in the sense of a complex sequence of predictable

acts, resulting in some predetermined desirable end product. Nursing is, we believe, processual, in the sense that it is always unfolding and that it is guided by intention. To characterize nursing situations with a nursing diagnosis and to portray the situation as a linear process driven by diagnosis or problem to be addressed with a pre-envisioned outcome would be to rob the situation of all the beauty of nursing. (p. 30)

The nurse responds to each call for nursing in a way that represents the uniqueness of the nurse and her/his own expressions of caring. Each response to a particular nursing situation would be slightly different and would portray the beauty of the nurse as caring person. It is in this way that the art of nursing is created by each nurse in each situation. Sharing this art deepens our understanding of the richness of our practice and provides an opportunity to reflect on the range of knowledge essential to expert nursing care. The following nursing situation, *Where Are They Now*, was created by one of our RN to BSN students. This is an example of a situation which could be used in class to study the nursing of persons who are dying.

Where Are They Now?

Jaime Castaneda, BSN

Hello my friend, my dying friend.
There you lie, an old man, weak and all alone
resting in a bed of thoughts, staring back in time,
gasping for every bit of life you have left,
with no one here to ease your moment but me, your nurse.
I wonder who hides behind such hopeless look and blank stare.
Were you a crying baby once introduced into this world
by a proud mother,
who showered you with hugs and kisses, hopes and dreams?
Or perhaps a playful child full of energy and imagination
who would grow up to become a teenager in love?
Were you someone's brother, husband, or maybe even a father?
Did you have any friends?
Where is everybody now? Does anybody care?
As we've come to meet, I watch death take you away
and the light within you subsides.
Each breath becomes weaker, and each pulse an eternity.
The moment freezes in time as darkness engulfs your light.

Thus, I watch you being absorbed.
Yet, there is nobody else here but me, your nurse,
to ease your path, share your moment,
hear your silent cry, and bring hope to those hopeless eyes.
The hope that you are not alone, and
that behind the darkness there is a light.
Somehow we've come to meet, as the
writings of your life come to an end,
the terminal lines of your final chapter
become the introductory ones of mine
Your past, unknown to me,
for the mystery of life is yours to keep.
I witness the pages of your past vanish deep
into your memory and become part of your soul.
Your present, I've come to meet.
An old man dying quietly in a hospital bed,
illuminated by the dim light of a sealed window,
and in the absence of fresh air for your soul to fly away.
Surrounded by an empty room filled with loneliness, and
crowded with memories, with nobody else here but me, your nurse.
Allow me to share this moment with you
and bridge your passage into that new place of endless dreams,
where love, energy and playfulness reign.
Where those arms, that once proudly introduced you into this world,
are anxiously waiting for you,
to shower you again with hugs and kisses, hopes and dreams.
My friend, my old, dying friend.
I wish you could see that you are not alone
and hear my thoughts of you, the patient, the child, the man.
As I contemplate your life for what it might have been
and offer my friendship, hoping to illuminate the way
to your death with my presence, my true presence.
Good bye my friend.

Students studying this nursing situation might reflect on the following questions:

- Who is the nurse as caring person?
- Who is the person nursed as caring person?
- How is the nurse expressing caring in this moment?

- How might the student's personal knowing or study of the dying experience influence knowledge necessary to understand the nursing situation?

- What empirical knowledge is essential to hear the calls and create responses that nurture wholeness through caring in this situation (e.g., approaches to being-with and communication guided by nursing theories, imminent signs of death, pain assessment and treatment, evidence-based practice protocols and nursing research about care of dying persons, and research questions that might be generated related to spiritual caring, presence, and touch)?

- What ethical knowing is inherent in this situation if nursing is practiced from the perspective of caring? What ethical dilemmas present in care of persons at the end of life and what ethical frameworks would be useful in guiding responses?

- What kind of healing environment ought to be created for dying persons?

- What are the possibilities for growth and nurturance of personhood in this situation?

- What are the hoped-for outcomes of nursing care?

As the nursing situation is retold and relived, nursing knowledge emerges and is developed and shared; nursing research knowledge and evidence-based practice guidelines are discussed; questions for research are generated; students and faculty members grow in their understanding of caring and caring relationships; and the richness of nursing as a discipline and practice emerges. Studying nursing in this way assists students in developing and celebrating nursing knowledge. They grow in their substantive understanding of caring and their appreciation of caring as nursing's unique contribution to the health and wholeness of persons.

Knowledge from prerequisite and supporting courses in the program of study such as pathophysiology, pharmacology, assessment, technical skills, literature, or psychology is brought to the study of the nursing situation as part of the range of knowledge necessary to hear calls and design nursing responses. This approach appropriately uses content from other disciplines to understand and practice nursing. However, as Touhy states, "while nurses respond to sequelae of illness, these responses should not take precedence over care of persons" (2004, p.45). Emphasis in nursing courses is on critical reflection and integration of knowledge in specific nursing situations, and creation of nursing responses. The study of caring is integral to knowing nursing and is a focus in each nursing course at all levels of the program. The study of caring requires critical reading of meaningful substantive literature, reflection, dialogue, and incorporation into thoughtful practice (Schoenhofer, 2001).

Nursing situations are clustered within courses based on traditional and social expectations. In the undergraduate program, particular nursing situations from a common setting are grouped by course (i.e., *Nursing Situations in Community, Nursing Situations in Psychiatric and Mental Health Care, Nursing Situations in Practice: Caring for Adults Experiencing Acute Alterations in Health*). In the undergraduate Nursing Research course, students reflect on a nursing situation experienced in their practice as the foundation for a paper exploring evidence-based practice and nursing research related to questions arising from the nursing situation. In the culminating undergraduate course, students study nursing situations within organizational structures that influence the nurturing of wholeness and well-being of persons and the environment.

In the masters program, students study nursing situations experienced by nurses at the advanced practice level in a variety of settings depending on the designated major focus or track chosen by the student. Nursing education majors study nursing education in a caring-based curriculum, nursing administration and clinical nurse leader majors focus on the creation of health-care environments grounded in caring, and nurse practitioner students study caring in nursing situations in primary care and with clients of all ages, depending on the focus.

The College has two doctoral programs: the Doctor of Philosophy (PhD) and the Doctor of Nursing Practice (DNP). Students in the PhD program focus on the development of caring knowledge through research and theory development. Each PhD dissertation contributes to the growth of caring science. DNP students focus on transforming systems of care that reflect caring values in their roles as nurse practitioners or nurse administrators. Curriculum plans for all programs of study are accessible at http://nursing.fau.edu/index.php?main=2&nav=294 on the College Web site.

Nursing practice courses provide undergraduate and graduate students with the opportunity to experience nursing situations in a full range of practice settings. Course objectives parallel those of the lecture course and are derived from the same themes. Faculty members, students, and preceptor nurses share in the teaching and learning process. Reflection and dialogue about the nursing situations experienced provide the opportunity to grow in the understanding of nursing as nurturing the wholeness of persons through caring.

EVALUATION OF CARING IN PRACTICE

A question often asked is how does one evaluate the professionalization of caring. In the undergraduate program, a Collaborative Nursing Practice Evaluation Tool organized around Roach's "6Cs" (1987) of compassion, competence, confidence, conscience, commitment, and comportment is used for student self-evaluation and faculty and preceptor evaluation of the student. Each of the "Cs" has been operationalized into expected competencies that students must demonstrate at an acceptable level. Table 9.2 provides an example of outcome indicators of conscience.

Students rate themselves on a numerical scale on each of the competencies, and the faculty and preceptor also rate the student both at mid-term and at the end of the semester. From the "6Cs," 12 critical

TABLE 9.2   Caring Competencies and Outcome Indicators

CARING COMPETENCIES AND OUTCOME INDICATORS	MIDTERM RATING	FINAL RATING
Conscience: The morally sensitive self attuned to values and integral to personhood	Self:	Self:
	Faculty:	Faculty:

- Plans care in partnership with patient, honors human dignity, and respects patient's rights and choices.
- Demonstrates accountability for own actions.
- Analyzes ethical and legal issues in each nursing situation.
- Supports fairness and nondiscrimination in health care.
- Demonstrates professional caring by considering how to influence systems and policies impacting health care.
- Demonstrates role of the nurse as advocate in the nursing situation.
- Always plans for continuity of care, effectively teaches patients and families.

behaviors have been selected, which students must complete at a satisfactory level.

The evaluations of graduate students in practicum courses also reflect caring competencies for advanced practice nursing, administration, education, or the clinical nurse leader role and are conducted collaboratively with the students, preceptors, and faculty members. Graduate students are expected to journal weekly on their experiences, reflecting on how they came to know the person nursed and how they integrated ways of knowing in hearing and responding to calls for nursing. They also prepare a written or oral presentation of a nursing situation.

PEDAGOGICAL PRACTICES

Pedagogical approaches to the study of nursing reflect the faculty's perspective of the discipline and their beliefs about learning. The philosophy states that a "supportive environment for learning is a caring environment. A caring environment is one in which all aspects of the human person are respected, nurtured, and celebrated. The learning environment emphasizes collegial relationships with faculty and students" (Christine E. Lynn College of Nursing, 2005). The Dance of Caring Persons is the model for the study of nursing. In the dance are faculty members, students, administrators, colleagues, the community, and the nursed. Each dancer is committed to the study of the discipline of nursing with caring as a central domain of knowledge. A culture of living caring encourages dialogue, debate, and appreciating different ways of knowing for faculty members and students. Teaching and learning occur through open dialogue and reflection rather than in a lecture format where facts and principles are presented.

The focus on the study of the nursing situation is on the person(s) nursed and how the caring between the nurse and one nursed nurtures wholeness. This is different from the common approach of teaching nursing through a review of diseases, symptoms, and interventions. Students and faculty members bring their breadth and depth of knowledge and experience to this study and learn from and with each other. Faculty members are not expected to have all the answers; reflection on each unique nursing situation uncovers and discovers the range of calls and possible nursing responses.

Nursing situations studied in class represent the actual lived experience of students and nurses in nursing practice settings. They may come from the experience of the faculty member or the student and may be presented in various art forms. Students are encouraged to reflect on the uniqueness and beauty of their nursing situations and represent through some aesthetic form. These aesthetic projects, integrated through all programs of study, illustrate through deep reflection the caring expressed in a nursing situation. Following is a representation of a nursing situation by graduate student Patricia LaMedica.

Human Tide

Together as birth waters broke
Together as your tide recedes
Solid earth moving under waves
Here, riding out this last bit of your storm
Between the living and the dying we touch
Mother-Daughter
Nursed-Nurse
You are slipping away
Like so many grains of sand in my hand
I need you to stay
I whisper for you to go
Oh, your ragged breath
The heaving of your body
In and out
Hypnotic swells that rise and fall
Rogue wave rises up and crashed upon the shore
Angry foam rushes in, swiftly recedes
Your life water whisked away
Leaves me bereft upon the shore.

Other examples of aesthetic representations can be found in *Nightingale Songs* (http://nursing.fau.edu/index.php?main=1&nav=475). Through the study of nursing situations, students continually focus on who they are as caring persons in a particular nursing situation and how the caring between the participants enhances personhood and nurtures wholeness for both the nurse and person nursed. Through the study of nursing situations, students learn to conceptualize, reflect, think critically, come to know self and others as caring, value and respect person, and ground nursing responses in caring.

Nursing practice course expectations include care maps, weekly reflective journals, facilitated dialogue, and simulated learning. Care maps are completed in undergraduate nursing practice courses. They invite the student to tell the story of the one nursed, identify knowledge needed to practice in this situation using multiple ways of knowing, reflect on self and other as caring person, identify calls for nursing, nursing responses, and evaluative data. These care maps are used instead of a traditional care plan based on the nursing process. The intent is to foster knowing of the one nursed as caring person.

Reflective journaling provides students the opportunity to appreciate the beauty of the nursing experiences they have encountered. Here is one example of a set of questions used in reflection:

- What are the calls for nursing?
- What possible nursing responses might be considered?
- Who is this person as caring person?
- How does this person live caring day to day?
- What is it like for me as student to be in this situation?
- How has reflection on the nursing situation enhanced my knowledge of nurturing the wholeness of person through caring?

Excerpt from a student's reflective journal:

As I walked into C.J.'s room, I was struck by the contrasting images of a seemingly healthy boy hooked up to so many different machines. Pictures of him, his family and his girlfriend scattered around the room like glimpses of a distant memory, C.J. lay in his bed, almost as if waiting to be woken up by his mom before school. As I approached his bed, he began to convulse in the way that my nurse preceptor had warned me he might. As I watched him, I was moved by the necessity of the caring philosophy in such a time as this. Medically, there was little we could offer C.J. as he was on the proper medications and receiving the appropriate treatment. A student nurse trained in the holistic care of persons, I suddenly realized there was something I could offer him: my authentic presence. Although C.J. was unable to communicate effectively with us, he was still a person complete in that moment and as his student nurse, I was committed to nursing his whole person. Thus, I turned on his cooling blankets, sat by his side and spoke with him. I told him how important he was to the nurses here and how I could tell how important he was to his family and friends without even meeting them. Our conversation may have been one sided verbally, but somehow I feel that he knew what I was saying to him and it made a therapeutic difference in the large picture enveloping our young man. (Marissa Bradford, undergraduate student)

The Blackboard Web-based course platform is used successfully for engaging students in discussions of living caring in nursing practice and articulation of how patterns of knowing were integrated into their study of nursing situations. This format allows all students in the course to share their learning, growth, and insights and learn from each other. Presentation of a nursing situation that has been experienced during the course and postconference discussions about nursing situations experienced are also utilized to enhance learning. In postconference discussions, students share the response to the direct invitation to care (inviting the nursed to help them come to know what matters most to them) (Boykin & Schoenhofer, 2001, p. 59), the range of knowledge necessary to come to know the person nursed and respond to calls and design responses, the hoped-for outcomes, and their understanding of the mutuality of the caring between.

Simulation is an integral part of practice learning. In each of the courses in the undergraduate program, and several in the master's program, faculty members have created scenarios that are staged in the simulation lab or virtual Lynn hospital with the Laerdal human patient simulators. These scenarios are developed to engage students in hearing and responding to calls for nursing that include competent performance of technical skills, assessment, and decision making regarding changes in a patient's vital signs, or providing authentic presence and touch during a time of anguish or fear. Faculty members or graduate teaching assistants assume the roles of family members and other health professionals as the scenario is enacted so that students respond to the totality of a dynamic situation. In the debriefing following enactment of the scenario, students are asked to reflect on the calls for nursing presented in the situation and how their responses reflected Roach's 6 Cs (1987), Mayeroff's (1971) caring ingredients, or concepts from Nursing as Caring (Boykin & Schoenhofer, 2001), or other theories. In this way, students are engaged in reflecting on the salience of caring knowledge to their practice.

ADVANCING CARING THROUGH RESEARCH, PRACTICE, AND SERVICE

With the mission, vision, and values of the College grounded in caring, the centrality of caring goes beyond the teaching mission and the educational programs of the College to infuse the research, practice, and service missions as well.

Caring and the Research Mission

The research mission of the College of Nursing is advancing the body of knowledge of caring in the discipline of nursing. This mission is realized through the organizational structure, faculty recruitment, and a mentoring program for new faculty members. The College of Nursing has an Office of Research and Scholarship whose purpose is to support faculty members in advancing their programs of research. This Office has an Associate Dean for Research and Scholarship and two research administrators who support faculty members in preparing grants and in post-award grant management. A well-funded intramural grants program exists to support pilot work with the expectation that this work will lead to proposals for external funding. The criteria for awarding this intramural funding include the development of an explicit connection to advancing caring knowledge. The guidelines for applicants state, "How does the proposed work emerge from a caring philosophy and fit into your ongoing research program?" Caring knowledge can be conceptualized as particular caring theories or explicit philosophical values that are common to a variety of theoretical perspectives. It is the responsibility of the researcher to establish the connection between their work and the advancement of caring science; in this way, the College encourages faculty members to shape their research trajectories within a caring framework.

Faculty recruitment is influenced by the caring values of the College. When prospective faculty members apply for positions, interview questions include queries about their understanding and appreciation of the philosophy and how they view their work within the context of advancing caring knowledge. These questions offer prospective faculty members the opportunity to be reflective and intentional in their choice to join our community. The goal of pursuing research and making scholarly contributions to the body of knowledge related to caring in nursing is understood. For example, new faculty members are pursuing research programs related to disruptive behavior (horizontal violence) in the workplace and its relationship to nurse retention and patient safety; what matters most to carers of people with mild to moderate dementia; implementing and evaluating *Nursing as Caring* (Boykin & Schoenhofer, 2001) as a model guiding nursing practice on an acute care unit; enhancing cancer screening in underserved minority populations; and understanding the experiences of adolescents who injure themselves by cutting. In each of these diverse research projects, the faculty members have made some explicit relationship to caring values and advancing caring science.

Each new faculty member enters a structured mentoring program designed individually to transition the faculty member into this College culture of caring. The program involves engagement of the faculty member with a mentorship team. The team consists of senior faculty members who focus on the new faculty member's growth in all three missions and who can guide the faculty member toward success. Research mentors help new faculty members identify an initial trajectory including sources of funding. Faculty members' growth is nurtured by the Associate Dean for Research and the research mentors; they support the development of manuscripts, identify opportunities for faculty development in key areas through attendance at educational programs, and guide the faculty members in grant-writing. Faculty members are oriented to the College of Nursing philosophy including the salient literature related to caring. Monthly dialogues on integrating caring into teaching are held, and new faculty members are encouraged to attend. New faculty members are connected with more senior faculty members who may be working in related areas. Currently there are four major research focus areas in the College: promoting healthy aging, evaluating integrative approaches to care, reducing health disparities, and transforming environments of care. All four of these focus areas have a strong explicit relationship to advancing caring knowledge.

Caring and the Practice Mission

Although not identified as a mission distinctive from service, it is useful to focus on practice separately because of its importance to nursing as a professional discipline. The College has focused on its interrelationships with practice through the development of several centers and through partnerships with health-care organizations. Two centers in the College deliver care to the community. One is the Louis and Anne Green Memory and Wellness Center, whose unique mission is grounded in the College's philosophy of caring. "The mission of the Center is to meet the complex needs of persons with memory disorders and their families through a comprehensive array of services, compassionate and innovative programs of care, research and education" (http://nursing.fau .edu/index.php?main=6&nav=156). Noteworthy programs, such as caregiver support and art therapy, acknowledge the wholeness and inherent healing capacity of persons and families. The explicit intention of the Center is to "treat the whole person with dignity and respect, enabling each client to function at his or her personal best and to maximize his or her quality of life" (http://nursing .fau.edu/index.php?main=6&nav=156). The Center's building was specifically designed to house a diagnostic clinic, a dementia-specific adult day center, and counseling and educational and research activities. Baccalaureate, masters, and doctoral students in the College have practice experiences at the Center. In this way, students can witness and engage in nursing practice that reflects the College philosophy. The Center becomes a laboratory where caring is studied and lived.

The Center for Innovations in School and Community Well-Being is the umbrella for several nurse-managed community wellness centers that are based in or adjacent to schools in West Palm Beach and Delray Beach, with satellites at nearby schools and community agencies. An array of services, directed by advanced practice nurses and social workers in collaboration with other health-care providers are provided at these community locations within a nurturing environment, including primary care, school health services, immunizations, health screenings, teen clinics, health promotion, counseling, and referrals. The College has operated two nurse-managed Centers, one in Delray Beach and the second at Westgate in West Palm Beach.

The Diabetes Education and Research Center (DERC) is a freestanding Center funded and operated by the Palm Healthcare Foundation. The Center is directed by advanced practice nurses who are certified diabetes educators, in collaboration with specialists in pediatric and adult endocrinology, pharmacy, social work, podiatry, nutrition, and exercise. The College of Nursing focus on nursing as nurturing wholeness of persons and environments through caring grounds the care provided in the Center. Building on this foundation, the distinctive Community Nursing Practice Model that has been developed in FAU Community Wellness Centers over the past 10 years guides community and family-centered care for those who are referred to the Center. This Center offers community-based health education programs for children and adults and their families, with or at risk of diabetes or complications of the disease. Nurses and other health professionals provide individualized, family-centered programs on prevention of obesity and complications of diabetes as well as self-care management and overall health promotion to persons who are referred to the Center from physicians and other primary care providers. Community education programs of health promotion and disease prevention are provided in schools, churches, community, and residential centers (http://nursing.fau.edu/index.php?main=6&nav=159). Students in the College of Nursing have practicum experiences at the Delray and Westgate Centers and DERC. For example, students organize and implement a community health fair at the DERC; nurse practitioner students complete practicum experiences at the Westgate Center, and students in advanced health assessment conduct comprehensive assessments including the required physical examinations for preschool children at the Delray Center. In all these situations, students are able to practice in environments that are part of the College, explicitly reflecting its philosophy and values.

The Nursing Leadership Institute (NLI) was founded in 2002 to provide nurses with the knowledge they require to succeed in a wide range of health-care and educational settings. The NLI concept evolved from meetings with nurse executives in the area who expressed a need to prepare nurse leaders grounded in the essential values of nursing, with the complex knowledge needed to lead competently and compassionately. NLI educational programs are designed using research findings with nursing leaders. The goal is to help nurses to enhance their leadership skills in the workplace through continuing education programs and sharing of best practices. The Novice Nursing Leadership Institute (NNLI) was founded in 2006 to address the transition gap between nursing education and entry-level practice. The NLI's unique collegiate/community partnership is guided by discussions held regularly with nursing leaders from the South Florida Community at the Dean's Dialogue with Colleagues (http://nursing .fau.edu/index.php?main=6&nav=158).

The Initiative for Intentional Well-Being is located in the College of Nursing and offers programs related to holistic health. For example, yoga classes are offered 5 days a week; healing touch is available by appointment; Reiki classes are offered to nurses; and community meditation gatherings are held weekly. The purpose of the initiative is to integrate holistic caring practices into nursing education and practice.

Nursing education-practice partnerships have been created to transform practice environments through implementing caring-based practice models. For example, the Port St. Lucie Medical Center partnered with the College of Nursing to adopt Boykin and Schoenhofer's (2001) theory of Nursing as Caring as the model to guide care delivery for the entire organization. Several faculty members and students were involved in this project. Similarly, other hospitals have approached the College about the development of dedicated education units (DEUs) at their hospitals (Moscato, Miller, Logsdon, Weinberg, & Chorpenning, 2007). These units have a mission of creating an environment in the hospital setting that supports education of students and staff and nursing research. The DEU established in partnership with St. Mary's Hospital is unique in that the unit adopted Nursing as Caring (Boykin & Schoenhofer, 2001) as the practice model guiding care on the unit. A faculty member is the Project Director for the DEU; her salary is supported by both the College and the hospital. A clinical group of baccalaureate students is assigned to the DEU for most of their required practicum experiences. Nurses on the unit are selected to serve as nursing practice mentors; in this role they are affirmed as nurse experts, precepting students on the unit and testing the theory-guided practice model with the students. Graduate students are present on the unit for their teaching practica, capstone projects, and independent studies. This synergy creates the excitement of mutual commitment to and enthusiasm for practice-education partnerships in learning and creating shared environments that reflect caring values.

Caring in the Service Mission

Faculty members provide service to the local, state, national, and global communities that reflects the philosophy of the College. For example, several faculty members provide primary care to underserved communities in the geographic service area. Students participate in service learning by partnering with communities to complete projects that are priorities for these communities. Two faculty members provide service to a northern county in Florida by assessing community needs that can be addressed by school nurses. Several faculty members are serving as educators and consultants in Uganda, the Philippines, and Thailand related to caring education and practice models. Faculty members, students, and alumni immediately responded to the crisis in Haiti providing critically needed nursing services to a suffering island nation neighbor to South Florida.

LOOKING TO THE FUTURE

Several trends affirm the directions taken by our College in building a school dedicated to caring: advancing the science, practicing the art, studying its meaning, and living it day to day. One indicator is that hospitals on the journey toward magnet status designation or those with magnet status (http://www.nursecredentialing.org/Magnet.aspx) must articulate a theoretical framework that guides nursing practice. Caring frameworks have been adopted by many hospitals; several in South Florida and other areas of the country are using Nursing as Caring (Boykin & Schoenhofer, 2001) as a model for practice. Others have contacted the College for consultation in transforming their practice environments through a caring-based approach to nursing practice. Educational-practice partnerships are the logical way to bridge the practice-education gap through transforming practice environments and educating students in real practice laboratories directed by caring theories.

Another example of this growth in interest in bringing Caring Science into the nursing workplace is the Watson Caring Science Institute (www.watsoncaringscience.org) and the consortium of hospitals guided by Watson's theory of human caring (http://www.watsoncaringscience.org/icc/index.html). These organizations provide evidence of a movement to change the current health-care environment to reflect values of compassion, relationship, and creating healing environments.

Next, the recent Carnegie Report (Benner, Sutphen, & Leonard, 2010) on the future of nursing education calls for reforms that have been foundational to the caring-based approach to education within the Christine E. Lynn College of Nursing. This report calls for a situated, contextual approach to learning through the use of narratives, patient interviews, and case studies that engages students in clinical reasoning and clinical imagination. They recommend greater attention to the integration of theory and practice in both classroom and clinical settings. This is consistent with the use of nursing situations in both classroom and clinical learning in clinical conferences. The nursing curricula of the College build upon a strong foundation in arts, humanities, and the sciences and integrate this knowledge, including aesthetics, into learning. Increasing the use of simulation is another recommendation; we have been developing simulations that reflect caring values and provide opportunities for students to integrate caring knowledge within practice. This unique approach to simulation transforms it from an exercise in technical know-how and critical thinking to a rehearsal of ethical comportment and growing ontological competencies (Watson, 1999) so important to living caring in practice situations.

Finally, the College has established the Archives of Caring in Nursing with the mission of preserving the history of Caring in Nursing, inviting the study of Caring, advancing Caring as an essential domain of nursing knowledge, and creating meaning for the practice of nursing. Descriptions and indexes to the collections are accessible on the College's Web site at http://nursing.fau.edu/index.php?main=6&nav=536. We are committed to securing the papers of Caring scholars and developing and maintaining the Archives to provide access to primary sources. This preserves the caring knowledge of the past as a springboard for knowledge development for the future.

It is evident that the Christine E. Lynn College of Nursing has laid the foundation for the future. The focus on caring is a part of the organizational structure and culture. It is reflected in the mission, vision, values, and philosophy and is explicitly present in curricular themes, program, and course objectives. The culture of living caring is strong, and as in any culture, it will endure with mentoring and orientation programs.

Our doctoral program focuses on knowledge development in caring. With this emphasis we are establishing a future for the advancement of Caring Science. Those prepared at the doctoral level will bring their research program and the values and approaches to knowledge development underpinning it to other schools of nursing, seeding and growing these ideas in other locations.

With an increasing number of national and international nursing scholars studying caring, we are considering alternative educational models that can be offered to those who want to study caring. This could be in the form of a certificate program or an Institute for Caring Studies. Sustaining a caring-based program across time will take a committed group of scholars, continuous reflection on the mission of the College, and consistent community building and outreach. For those of us who believe that the work is essential for the future of the discipline of nursing and the lives of those we nurse, it is a labor of love.

REFERENCES

Benner, P., Sutphen, M., Leonard, V., & Day, L. (2010). *Educating nurses: A call for radical transformation* (Carnegie Foundation for the Advancement of Teaching. Preparation for the Professions Program). San Francisco: Jossey-Bass.

Boykin, A. (Ed.). (1994). *Living a caring-based program*. New York: National League for Nursing Press.

Boykin, A., & Schoenhofer, S. (2001). *Nursing as caring*. Boston: Jones and Bartlett.

Cameron, J. (1992). *The artist's way*. New York: Putnam & Sons.

Carper, B. (1978). Fundamental patterns of knowing in nursing. *Advances in Nursing Science, 1,* 13–24.

Christine E. Lynn College of Nursing. (2005). *The philosophy.* Retrieved from http://nursing.fau.edu:8082/exchweb/bin/redir.asp?URL=http://nursing.fau.edu/newnursingsite/philosophy.html, http://nursing.fau.edu/index.php?main=1&nav=635

Easwaran, E. (1989). *The compassionate universe: The power of the individual to heal the environment*. Tomales, CA: Nilgiri Press.

Leininger, M. (1981). *Caring: An essential human need*. Thorofare, NJ: Slack.

Mayeroff, M. (1971). *On caring*. New York: Harper and Row.

Moscato, S. R. Miller, J., Logsdon, K., Weinberg, S., & Chorpenning, L. (2007). Dedicated education unit: An innovative clinical practice education model. *Nursing Outlook, 55,* 31–37.

Paterson, J., & Zderad, L. (1976). *Humanistic nursing*. New York: John Wiley Biomedical Publication.

Roach, S. (1987). *The human act of caring*. Ottawa, ON: Canadian Hospital Association.

Rogers, M. (1970). *An introduction to the theoretical basis of nursing*. Philadelphia: FA Davis.

Schoenhofer, S. (2001). Infusing the nursing curriculum with literature on caring: An idea whose time has come. *International Journal for Human Caring, 5*(2), 7–14.

Simon, S. B., & Clark, J. (1975). *More values clarification: strategies for the classroom*. San Diego, CA: Pennant Press.

Touhy, T. (2004). Dementia, personhood and nursing: Learning from a nursing situation. *Nursing Science Quarterly, 17*(1), 43–49.

Touhy, T., & Boykin, A. (2008). Caring as the central domain in nursing education. *International Journal for Human Caring, 12*(2), 8–15.

Watson, J. (1979). *Nursing: The philosophy and science of care*. Boston: Little, Brown.

Watson, J. (1999). *Post modern nursing and beyond*. New York: Churchill Livingstone.

Ustal, D. (1977). Searching for values. *Image, 9*(1), 15–17.

10
Caring-Human Science Philosophy in Nursing Education: Beyond the Curriculum Revolution

SHEILA LEWIS, MHSc, BScN, CHTP
MARTHA ROGERS, EdD, MScN, RN
RAHEL NAEF, MN, RN

T HIS PAPER DESCRIBES THE EVOLUTION of a nursing curriculum based on the work of Bevis and Watson (1989, 2000), and illustrates how it has expanded into one that explicitly includes an understanding of nursing as a human science. The "Caring-Human Science Curriculum" entails a particular emphasis on trans-theoretical integration, whereby multiple nursing theories consistent with the curriculum's philosophy are embraced. Unique characteristics of the curriculum are illustrated, and faculty and students' experiences of teaching and learning processes are discussed. This paper concludes by addressing some of the insights gained from living the "Caring-Human Science Curriculum" for nursing education.

Nearly a decade and a half ago, Bevis and Watson (1989) startled nursing education with their provocative book, Toward a Caring Curriculum: A New Pedagogy for Nursing. The authors clearly stated that the purpose of the work was "to create a new curriculum-development paradigm for nursing education" (p. 1). Offering a critical

Reprinted with permission from Lewis, S., Rogers, M., & Naef, R. (2006). Caring-human science philosophy in nursing education: Beyond the curriculum revolution. *International Journal for Human Caring, 10*(4), 31–37.

appraisal of the dominant behaviorist paradigm in nursing education, they argued for a shift in the pedagogy to one that embraced process, relationships of equity between teachers and learners, and the total reconceptualization of learning. The aim was to humanize the educational process in a way that fostered individuality, creativity, and the legitimization of multiple modes of knowing as sources of experience and learning. The work of Bevis and Watson catalyzed what has since been called the nursing curriculum revolution.

As a program that embraced the "Caring Curriculum," we have now had the experience of living and evolving with the new paradigm for a decade. We have achieved significant changes to the curriculum and to the processes of teaching-learning. We have witnessed the experiences of students, teachers, and graduates. We have stumbled, questioned, and struggled with our own competing paradigms and ways of being yet we persist in our belief that the curriculum revolution is necessary if we are to educate in a way that is consistent with the philosophy we seek to teach our students. In this paper, we will set out the philosophical underpinnings of our curriculum and discuss how the curriculum has evolved from the "Caring Curriculum" to the "Caring-Human Science Curriculum." Informed by our experiences, we will discuss our assumptions, values, and beliefs in relation to how they are lived in the teaching-learning processes, as well as the challenges of living the "Caring Human Science Philosophy" in nursing education.

EMANCIPATION FROM BEHAVIORISM

Tyler (1949) is attributed with the creation of the behaviorist model of education, a model embraced across many fields and disciplines including nursing. Nurse educators embraced this model because the assumptions, values, and beliefs seemed very consistent with those of the dominant biomedical model and the Cartesian world-view. There was a kinship of sorts.

From the perspective of the Tylerian model, learning is conceptualized as a linear, systematic process involving assessment of learning needs, objective formulation, content development, delivery to the students, and evaluation. The emphasis is placed on performance, where educators objectively determine the gap between actual and desired performance and design a program to meet the apparent deficits. Evaluation is based on goal attainment that must be objectively measured. Learning, from this point of view, is considered to be instrumental where each new learning experience is viewed as building incrementally on existing knowledge and skill (Mezirow, 1990).

"The basic assumption of the behaviorist model is that it is possible to predict, fairly accurately, the outcomes of instruction" (Bevis, in Bevis & Watson, 2000). Objectivity, efficiency, and rationality are the consequences of this view. It follows then that from the behaviorist perspective the teacher is seen as the expert and transmitter of knowledge, with the learner as a passive object to be filled with information. Bevis and Watson acknowledged that a behaviorist approach to teaching and learning "is excellent for those aspects of curriculum that are oriented toward memorization and skills. Its misuse has come in trying to make it uniformly applicable to all nursing curriculum matters, and in limiting curriculum exploration to the behaviorist theory" (p. 3).

There is little doubt that the Tylerian model lives on, either consciously or unconsciously, in the minds of many. One needs only to look at hospital-based orientation or in-service education programs for nurses to clearly see evidence of behaviorism. The competency-based approaches to education and the reductionistic specification of professional practice or accreditation standards are reflective of this model. Further, behaviorism continues to thrive as the basis of many nursing curricula today. It is extraordinarily difficult to break free from a paradigm that has dominated for decades and particularly one that has had such a strong affinity to the natural science worldview. Questioning behaviorist pedagogy means questioning more than teaching. It means questioning fundamental assumptions about human beings, relationships, nursing, learning, and the meaning of truth and reality.

HUMANISTIC-EDUCATIVE CARING PARADIGM

With the introduction of the humanistic-educative caring paradigm as the pedagogical framework for nursing education, Bevis and Watson (1989, 2000) challenged educators to consider an alternative to behaviorist model. In contrast with the positivistic assumptions of the behaviorist model, the humanistic-educative caring model assumes that curriculum is really about process; the interactions and transactions that occur between and among learners and teachers where there is an intent for learning to occur (Bevis & Watson, 2000). From this perspective, learning is not limited to the intellectual realm; rather, it is a whole human experience, one that may affect the mind, heart, body, and soul. Wholeness of the learning experience can foster self-insight and growth, creativity, artistry, and imagination merging in the development of scholarship. The humanistic-educative caring paradigm assumes that learning is not a linear process the outcomes of which cannot fully be determined a priori. Learning is an unfolding journey of meaning-making that is unique for each learner. Learning is facilitated in an environment that is caring and respectful, and where students believe they are safe to express their questions, ideas, or emerging thoughts. Students learn about creative critical thinking and the never-ending possibilities of human potential.

The humanistic-educative caring paradigm embraces openness to possibility and to the relativity of truth:

> Teaching is knowledge beyond the given. It is allegorical knowing, knowing of the possibility of a situation, of the potentiality of the child, of the manner in which this potentiality may be actualized, the ways in which its logos may be brought to our presence . . . Teaching, then, like art, is making the way open for the Being of beings to unconceal itself as truth— which, after all, is what teaching is all about. When authentic, teaching is a mode of being through which unconcealedness— that is, truth—takes place. (Goetz, 1983, in Bevis, 2000, p. 217)

Bevis (2000) speaks to the notion of learning as the "unconcealment" of truth, not through traditional "telling" but through "opening a way or seeing the possibilities of a situation" (p. 217). Dewey (1998), a distinguished educational philosopher, encouraged the cultivation of reflective thinking for the unconcealment of truth through open-mindedness, whole-heartedness, and responsibility. In order to see these possibilities in teaching-learning it is necessary to be committed to reflective thinking and ways of being that support the unconcealment of truth in all of its colors.

The humanistic-educative paradigm embraces openness to possibility. From the perspective of Bevis and Watson (2000), the humanistic-educative caring paradigm calls for a belief of teaching-learning as a process of human discovery where teachers and learners are coparticipants in the uncovering of meaning. It is a process that is open to possibility and that leads to the release of creativity, artistry, and scientific and theoretical imagination. Learning is fostered in a climate that embraces flexibility, dialogue, and deep reflection, as well as authentic caring and respect for each person's unique capacity for meaning-making, self-discovery, and knowledge creation.

EVOLUTION TOWARD THE "CARING-HUMAN SCIENCE CURRICULUM"

Nursing education evolves in tandem with the evolution of both society and nursing as a profession and discipline. Similarly, our curriculum has evolved over the last 10 years to one we now describe as the "Caring-Human Science Curriculum." The curriculum embraces our roots in the humanistic-educative caring paradigm, as well as Watson's earlier work on "caring" (Watson, 1999). However, it has evolved to incorporate more recent discourse in the area of human science-informed nursing theory. The curriculum addresses society's call for more holistic conceptions of health, concern for the natural environment, and for participatory relationships in caring-healing processes.

The "Caring-Human Science Curriculum" suggests a view of nursing that is reflective of what Parse (1987) has called the simultaneity paradigm and what Watson (1999, 2005) has called the unitary-transformative/unitary science paradigm. This view is philosophically informed by the human science tradition (Critchley, 2002; Dilthey, 1988; Polkinghorne, 1988). Transpersonal caring science (Watson) is one theoretical expression of a human science–based curriculum. However, the curriculum also embraces all nursing theoretical perspectives that are philosophically consistent with human science, such as those espoused by Parse (1981, 1995, 1997, 1998), Newman (1994, 1997), Rogers (1970, 1986, 1990), and others. The curriculum, then, expresses nursing as being philosophically based in the human sciences.

Recently, Watson and Smith (2002) suggested that it is time to consider the possibility of trans-theoretical integration of human science-based nursing theories. Illustrating the point, they discussed the integration of transpersonal caring science (Watson & Smith) with the science of unitary human beings (Rogers, 1986, 1990) by identifying commonalities yet still preserving the uniqueness of each. Smith (1999, 2004) further elaborated the discussion on the unitary worldview and trans-theoretical integration. This work captures, in a theoretical way, the organic evolution of our curriculum as it has evolved over the decade. By way of illustration, the following tenets, synthesized from the work of Newman (1994, 1997), Parse (1981, 1995, 1997, 1998),

Rogers (1970, 1986, 1990), and Watson (Watson, 1999, 2002), are central to the "Caring-Human Science Curriculum" as it is now emerging.

CENTRAL TENETS OF THE "CARING-HUMAN SCIENCE CURRICULUM"

1. Human beings are unitary beings, unique, whole, indivisible, and ever changing. Concepts: energy fields, consciousness, lived experience, and human becoming.
2. The environment is unitary; unique, whole, indivisible, infinite, and inseparable from human beings. Concepts: energy fields, consciousness is energy, human-universe process, human-environment field process, and global and universal field of consciousness.
3. Health and healing are processes, experienced and expressed uniquely. Concepts: energy fields, pattern, expanding consciousness, dynamic flow, and becoming as human-living-health.
4. Health and healing processes are manifestations of human emergence. Concepts: meaning, choosing, value priorities, transformation, transcendence with the possible, choice points, repatterning, creative emergence, and expanding consciousness.
5. Living, health and healing are boundaryless in space and time. Concepts: multidimensionally transcending, human-universe process, pandimensionality, universal consciousness, past-present-future, infinity, and pandimensional space-time.
6. Nurses are unitary beings in caring relationships with human beings living health and healing. Concepts: energy fields and graceful energy, caring consciousness, bearing witness, unconditional love, intentionality, multiple ways of knowing, and mutuality of transpersonal caring-healing relationship within caring field.
7. The relationships nurses have with human beings living health and healing are the essential purpose of nursing. Concepts: centering, true presence and authenticity, caring-healing relationship, life energy field/universal energy field, caring moment, transpersonal caring relationship, and search for meaning.
8. Transpersonal caring-healing modalities as healing arts and choices for transformation and self-healing by human beings. Concepts: "ethical relational, and energetic through caring

consciousness, intentionality, presence, authenticity; noninvasive, nonintrusive, natural-environmental healing modalities; those modalities that help to connect with universal field to access inner healer; intentional use of form, color, light, energy, sound, touch, visual, consciousness, etc." (Watson, 2005, p. 225).

The philosophical tenets and related nursing theoretical concepts illustrate the explicit paradigm that guides the curriculum in a way that embraces various nursing theories. In this way, the "Caring-Human Science Curriculum" encourages theoretical and method-ological pluralism yet retains a consistent perspective of nursing that is rooted in the human science worldview. Consequently, the curricu-lar evolution from the "Caring Curriculum" to the "Caring-Human Science Curriculum" has both deepened our commitment to nursing from a human science perspective while expanding in breadth toward greater inclusiveness for multiple nursing theoretical perspectives chosen by both faculty and students.

TEACHING AND LEARNING IN THE "CARING-HUMAN SCIENCE CURRICULUM"

The Caring-Human Science philosophy informs the content and focus of the curriculum, as well as pedagogical framework related to teaching and learning. What then might be the distinguishing characteristics of this curriculum? The following discussion aims to illuminate some of the unique features of the curriculum in terms of content and process.

Acquiring an Understanding of Nursing From a Nursing Perspective

Students come to understand the philosophical foundations of nursing and acquire an ability to understand and critically appraise the natural science and biomedical perspective vis a vis the human science perspective of nursing. As nursing knowledge is expressed through nursing theories, students learn about and practice in a way that is informed by one or more nursing theories that are consistent with human science paradigm. Students learn about theories and concepts derived from the natural sciences, as well as other fields and disciplines, while clearly understanding that nursing has its own distinct body of knowledge and unique perspective.

"Clinical Competence" and the Dance With Diverging Paradigms

Watson (1999) suggested that a unitary transformative paradigm is not only about epistemology. In fact, the proverbial proof in the pudding is related to the ontological shift the paradigm ought to catalyze. There is little doubt that one of the greatest challenges of living the "Caring-Human Science Curriculum" is that of considering the meaning of "clinical competence" from this perspective. We live and practice in environments that continue to strongly emphasize the natural science, biomedical paradigm. Moreover, there are high expectations for technical competence within the practice environments and among students themselves. Thus, there is a continuous push and pull in the dance of diverging paradigms.

The on-going challenge then is to help students acquire the clinical and technical skills that are required of them in practice and also to help them develop the "ontological competencies" (Watson, 1999) that are informed by the caring-human science perspective. We continue to evolve as we rise to this significant challenge of teaching-learning nursing as a discipline with a distinct and unique body of theoretical and empirical knowledge that informs nursing practice, and as a profession bound by standards and regulations embedded in current healthcare contexts (Parse, 1999).

Teaching students to learn to dance with diverging paradigms begins with what might be called paradigmatic awareness. Students are encouraged to examine the paradigm that is underlying the clinical and technical skills they are learning, that is, the discipline that underlies the profession or practice of nursing. This is not to juxtapose the biomedical and caring-human science paradigms in oppositional duality but rather to appreciate the dance of the two paradigms in the current practice realities. Developing awareness is essential if students are to learn how to dance with alternative paradigms.

Awareness alone will not enable students to learn to dance from their nursing perspective from the caring-human science paradigm. Students need to acquire deep knowledge of and facility with the steps, movement, and creative motions of their own dance. To do this, we begin by teaching students about the power of human relationships to heal, create, and transform.

Students develop the skill of being with another, openly and without judgment. They acquire the ability to fully listen (not just with ears) to the other as he/she expresses their experience and its meaning, and share their own knowledge of what they need, wish for, or imagine. Learning to be in a caring relationship and to respect and value persons' experiences of health and healing is the primary ontological competency from a caring-human science perspective. This ontological competency includes the clinical competency of listening openly and attentively to what persons have to say and to stay with them as they explore the meaning of their situation.

Students also acquire knowledge and skill in relation to a variety of other caring-healing modalities, depending upon the nursing theory that informs their practice. For instance, students may develop an understanding of the theory, skill, and art of touch, presencing, and listening. They may explore the physiological immunological evidence underpinning the back rub or the bath as healing acts rather than institutionally prescribed acts to complete. They may examine the research related to rocking as a healing motion and the incorporation of rocking into practice. They may explore the theoretical and scientific bases of healing touch, healing waters, movement or dance, music or poetry, and meditation or imagery. The ability of students to dance to their own tune depends on the acquisition of sound knowledge and competencies that are informed by the caring-human science paradigm.

The "Caring-Human Science Curriculum" means challenging conventional views of clinical competence. It is a difficult challenge because most of us, as faculty, learned to dance with the music of the biomedical model. Nevertheless, we move forward as choreographers of a new dance, one we hope will enable students to practice in a way that is philosophically, theoretically, and scientifically informed by nursing knowledge, espousing not only an expanded but also a different view of what constitutes clinical competency.

Toward Global Consciousness

The "Caring-Human Science Curriculum" embraces a fundamental belief in the unitary nature of the universe and all that is enfolded therein. This means that we understand the connectedness of all human beings to one another, as well as our integral relationship with our planetary home. While many, if not most, nursing programs teach about the community, our curriculum moves beyond community to explore the meaning of nursing in global health and healing. There is an explicit goal of fostering global consciousness and global citizenship through an exploration of the issues that face all humanity and the planet. Students may explore war and peace, pollution, the ozone layer, degradation of the rain forests, child labor, or poverty from a global perspective. They engage in critical analyses of values implicit in the Western cultural perspective with its emphasis on consumption and material wealth. They are also encouraged to extend their horizons to connect with past-present-future by exploring personal and collective histories as well as imagining the world of future generations. Consistent with our philosophical beliefs, students engage in learning that invites an exploration of the role of each student, as nurse and global citizen, in contributing to the health and well-being of humanity and planet, in both the present and the future.

Teaching-Learning Processes:
The Joy of the Noisy Classroom

Prospective students often ask what it is like to be a student in class. We explain that it is probably not what they imagine a class to be at a university. A stroll past classrooms in our program is likely to reveal students chattering, groups laughing, teams creating collages, dyads acting or dancing their interpretation of a nursing theory, or teachers joining students in creating a work of art. Generally, there is a palpable energy that exudes from the classroom. We have learned to appreciate the joy of the noisy classroom. The philosophic underpinnings of the "Caring-Human Science Curriculum" necessarily inform our understanding of teaching and learning. We understand learning as a process of human discovery rather than a product. Foremost, it is a communal enterprise whereby the collective quest to teach, learn, and to know about nursing, human beings, health, and healing nourishes the individual student in his/her personal learning and growing.

Teaching-learning is facilitated in an environment that is caring, respectful, and safe. Learning occurs through reciprocal caring relationships that may bring insight, creativity, meaning, and transformation. This process adopts a learner-centered learning approach to teaching versus a teacher-centered approach to learning. Within this reciprocal transpersonal caring relationship among students and between students and faculty, light-filled openings are created for making "sense" of information in relation to each learner's prior knowledge and whole being. Learning is a whole human experience that unfolds in unique patterns for each person.

In our curriculum, the notion of academic rigor takes on new and expanded meaning. Conventional interpretations of academic rigor are founded in a belief that performance, in this regard, is strictly intellectual,in a cognitive sense. However, if we believe that learning is more than a cognitive endeavoring, that it is a whole human experience, then both the expression of scholarship and academic rigor ought to be holistically construed. Certainly, we aim to help students acquire the skills associated with reading, critical analysis, synthesis, formal writing, and the abilities to orally discuss and debate. We also aim to foster the exploration of scholarship and its expression in myriad ways. While written tests, exams, and essays are used to "measure" learning, we also encourage expressions of learning through art, dance, music, song, poetry, pottery, story, photography, or other aesthetic means. Not only do students begin to appreciate an expanded view of nursing scholarship and its expression but they also learn that patients too may express their own experiences, learnings, hopes, and dreams through the limitless, creative capacities of the human being. Table 10. 1 includes some of our teaching-learning approaches that reflect this learning journey.

Teaching-learning in the "Caring-Human Science Curriculum" challenges faculty to think about and, often, reconceptualize notions about clinical competence, academic rigor, scholarship, and nursing practice that are truly consistent with the theoretical and philosophical roots of the discipline. There is no doubt that teaching-learning is a journey of discovery for faculty and students alike. For students, particularly those who are experienced registered nurses, the journey of learning can be punctuated with times of confusion as well as joyful insight, which are all hallmarks of significant learning that challenges fundamental beliefs and values about human beings, nursing, health, and universe. The following narrative conveys the learning process as lived by an experienced registered nurse student who had returned to university to complete her Bachelor of Science in Nursing (BScN) degree.

TABLE 10.1   Creating Light-Filled Openings for Learning That Reflect a Caring-Human Science Philosophy

Developing a transpersonal caring relationship	Show genuine interest in students and create an atmosphere for authentic caring within this learning experience:
	1. Learn names through group process; have groups choose their group name based on their collective
	2. Use principles of cooperative learning in small group and plenary; encourage autonomy and a sense of both individual and group responsibility for the learning process
	3. Develop mutual goals for learning that focus on success, individual, and group learning needs; learners participate in the development of course, group, and individual learning objectives
	4. Build confidence and encourage the expression of thoughts and feelings without judgment
	5. Facilitate independent and group problem solving through listening, respectful dialogue, and structured reflection
	6. Offer support and serve as a resource for students; help each learner to find personal meaning in learning experiences
	7. Stay within the frame of reference of the learner
Creating a caring-healing consciousness through intentionality and caritas/ love-centered energy field	1. Prior to each class, center and ground self with positive intentions for this group of learners and this time and space
	2. At the beginning and end of each class, spend time to center with class through brief meditation and imagery; involve the class in choosing and leading this process
	3. Remain flexible and open to the possibilities within the learning environment and within each learner. Let go of the need to control the teaching experience and instead move like a "leaf on water" with the learning being directed by the learner within the frame of reference of the course goals and objectives
	4. Share of yourself and your lived experiences with the intention of opening the space for learners to share of themselves, their values, and their own lived experiences
	5. Practice loving-kindness with a sense of reverence and sacredness for all that unfolds in the learning experience
	6. Cherish all ways of knowing and facilitate the unfolding of these ways of knowing within the learning process
	7. See the spirit-filled person within each learner and create a learning space for learners to share this with each other
	8. Facilitate opportunities for dialogue that connects our heads with our hearts and our hands; praxis as the basis for advancement of our caring-healing practices

Evaluation of learning	1. Evaluation is a process of "authentication" in that students do self-evaluations and faculty engage in series of experiences, observations, papers, projects, and accomplishments that authenticate their learning (Watson, J., personal communication, April 5, 2006)
	2. Develop clear, transparent guidelines for progression with processes that are negotiated with the learners and teacher. Evaluation evidences should match with the course learning objectives agreed upon. These processes will support self-growth, increasing self-awareness, and an evolving sense of congruence with expectations for professional practice
	3. Honor students' self-learning process, self-pacing and self-correcting throughout the learning process
	4. Assess learning using methods that reflect multiple epistemological approaches and ways of knowing
	5. Reassess if inconsistent or incongruent data
	6. Acknowledge and act on decisions and realities with students' involvement in decision-making process based on standards of practice, ethical guidelines, etc. (Watson, J., personal communication, April 5, 2006).

LIVING THE "CARING-HUMAN SCIENCE CURRICULUM": A STUDENT'S PERSPECTIVE

My participation in the "Caring-Human Science Curriculum" has been a very meaningful and rewarding learning experience. My learning endeavor was enriched by the program's collaborative teaching-learning philosophy and its strong commitment to nursing knowledge and theory as a guide for practice. My engagement with multiple nursing theories and their philosophical and paradigmatic roots has provided me with a transformed understanding of the nursing discipline. In particular, the human science perspective of nursing has fundamentally reshaped my understanding of nursing as a field of study with a unique body of knowledge that informs and is constituted by nursing scholarship, research, and practice. My learning about human science nursing theories and the ways this distinct perspective informs multiple dimensions of nursing, such as practice, teaching-learning, change, leadership, and research, has provided me with a sense of identity and purpose in my nursing endeavors, as well as a language to articulate my nursing knowledge and practices.

Having received my basic nursing education in a program that (a) promoted a functional and biomedical conceptualization of nursing, thereby building on knowledge from many different disciplines but scarcely on nursing's own knowledge base and (b) proposed that a good nurse is technically competent and a skilful clinical expert who performs a wide range of activities to achieve optimal health for the patient, I started my BScN program with many questions regarding how nursing distinguishes itself from other health professions and disciplines.

In the "Caring-Human Science Curriculum" teaching-learning was always a collaborative journey into the yet unfamiliar realms of nursing knowledge as articulated in nursing theory, practice, and research. In this journey toward knowing, my own experiences, thinking, and ways of engaging with the subject matter were as important as the theoretical content to be worked through. This working through involved individual and collaborative ways of learning, where understandings, ideas, questions, struggles, and new awareness could be shared in the classroom, teaching-learning self and others at the same time. This allowed for a deeper understanding of myself as a nurse in relation to nursing's social mandate to promote health, healing, and quality of life and to engage in relationships and ways of caring and providing nursing services that are meaningful for persons in need of nursing services.

My engagement with nursing-specific knowledge answered some profound questions I was carrying with me while also challenging my assumptions, values, and beliefs about nursing in general and about nursing practice in particular. To remain open and staying committed to new ways of thinking has not always been easy as many of my previous actions and ways of practicing nursing were put into question. In particular, I struggled to understand how different paradigmatic conceptualizations of nursing and, in particular, the use of different bodies of knowledge based in different disciplines can coexist in nursing practice. Therefore, to find my way with such newly gained knowledge and its implications for my ways of being a nurse and practicing nursing has required me to reflect, to drill deeper, to try to understand better what it means to revere human life and diverse ways of living, and to be and stay with persons who experience changes in their health and quality of life and who live intense and profound moments of struggling, questioning, and finding meaning.

It has challenged me to contemplate, change, or stay the same but most of all to grow as a person and a nurse. Moreover, it has provided me with a clear sense of what nursing is and has framed my thinking about nursing, health, and persons, informing my nursing practice and scholarship.

Thus, my participation in the "Caring-Human Science Curriculum" has provided me with a distinct body of nursing knowledge, which now guides my thinking and ways of being and practicing as a nurse. At times, studying, learning about, and gaining an understanding of the different nursing theories, as well as the philosophical differences between nursing theories rooted in the natural vis a vis the human sciences, was overwhelming. To gain a comprehension of how nursing theory informs nursing practice, how each theory is different or similar, and which one resonates most profoundly with my own values and beliefs required an intense engagement with theoretical thought in relation to myself as a nurse and a person. Even though the "Caring-Human Science Curriculum" puts forth a view of nursing as human science, it also explicitly embraces pluralism. This means that as a student, I had the freedom and the challenge to choose and work with a nursing theory that speaks to me, while also learning about others.

As my nursing knowledge base changed through my engagement with nursing as a human science and as a particular nursing theory surfaced as the one to guide my nursing endeavours, my way of living nursing practice and engaging in nursing scholarship changed as well. While I still perform nursing skills and enact clinical competencies, my focus is on the person, family, or community as the ones who know best what is important to them and what they need. My understanding of health and healing has expanded and moved beyond any preconceived notion of norms or measurable entities. My ways of being with persons have taken on new dimensions. My focus is on persons' experiences of health and illness and quality of life, and ways of caring and services that are meaningful for them. I live my nursing practice through seeking persons' perspective, listening to, and promoting the services persons say they want and need. Living the "Caring-Human Science Curriculum" has been an important and transforming learning experience that has shaped and formed the way I am thinking and living nursing.

CONCLUSION

For students, faculty, and graduates, living the "Caring-Human Science Curriculum" is exhilarating and tremendously challenging at the same time. It is exhilarating because there is a pervasive feeling of a community working together to advance a view of nursing that honors the unique knowledge and practice of our discipline, as well as nursing's glorious mission to humankind. It is exhilarating to push the boundaries of convention in nursing education and to foster the expression of human experience and nursing scholarship intellectually, artistically, aesthetically, creatively, and through all forms of knowing and being. However, living the curriculum is also tremendously challenging in environments that are steeped in the natural science worldview.

Closing words from a student who expresses so clearly the challenges of living the "Caring-Human Science Curriculum:"

It is time for nursing to reclaim its voice in the process of change and to embrace the possibilities for the future. Active participation in change is an opportunity for a rewarding journey of self-discovery and higher learning. It is often the road less traveled and until nurses feel empowered by the process of change, maintaining the status quo will prove to be the road that boasts the most traffic. (K. Nixon, personal communication, 2004)

Living the "Caring-Human Science Curriculum" is, in a sense, an experience of living the paradoxical struggles of colliding paradigms yet we persist in the belief that our efforts are guided by a commitment to the future of nursing as a profession and a discipline and the health and well-being of humanity and planet.

I shall be telling this with a sigh
Somewhere ages and ages hence:
Two roads diverged in a wood, and I—
I took the one less traveled by
And that has made all the difference

(Frost, 1920)

REFERENCES

Bevis, E. O. (2000). Teaching and learning: A practical commentary. In E. O. Bevis & J. Watson (Eds.), *Toward a caring curriculum: A new pedagogy for nursing* (pp. 217–260). Boston: Jones & Bartlett Publishers.

Bevis, E. O., & Watson, J. (1989). *Toward a caring curriculum: A new pedagogy for nursing.* New York: National League for Nursing.

Bevis, E. O., & Watson, J. (2000). *Toward a caring curriculum: A new pedagogy for nursing.* Boston: Jones & Bartlett Publishers.

Critchley, S. (2002). Introduction. In S. Critchley & R. Bernasconi (Eds.), *The Cambridge companion to Levinas.* Cambridge, UK: Cambridge University Press.

Dewey, J. (1998). Why reflective thinking must be an educational aim. In J. Dewey (Ed.), *How we think: A restatement of the relation of reflective thinking to the educative process* (pp. 18–34). New York: Houghton Mifflin Co.

Dilthey, W. (1988). *Introduction to the human science: An attempt to lay a foundation for the study of society and history.* (Original work published in 1923.) Detroit, MI: Wayne State University Press.

Frost, R. (1920). The road not taken. In R. Frost (Ed.), *Mountain interval.* Retrieved September 20, 2005, from http://www/bartleby.com/119/.

Goetz, I. L. (1983). Heidegger and the art of teaching. *Educational Theory, 33*(1), 1–9.

Mezirow, J. (1990). *Fostering critical reflection in adulthood: A guide to transformative and emancipatory learning.* San Francisco: Jossey-Bass.

Newman, M. (1994). *Health as expanding consciousness* (2nd ed.). Sudbury, MA: James & Bartlett.

Newman, M. (1997). Evolution of theory of health as expanding consciousness. *Nursing Science Quarterly, 10*(1), 22–25.

Parse, R. R. (1981). *Man-living-health: A theory of nursing.* New York: Wiley.

Parse, R. R. (1987). *Nursing science: Major paradigms, theories, and critiques.* Philadelphia: Saunders.

Parse, R. R. (Ed.). (1995). *Illuminations: The human becoming theory in practice and research.* New York: National League for Nursing.

Parse, R. R. (1997). The human becoming theory: The was, is, and will be. *Nursing Science Quarterly, 10*(1), 32–38.

Parse, R. R. (1998). *The human becoming school of thought: A perspective for nurses and other health professionals.* Thousand Oaks, CA: Sage.

Parse, R. R. (1999). Nursing: The discipline and the profession. *Nursing Science Quarterly, 12*(4), 275–276.

Polkinghorne, D. (1988). *Narrative knowing and the human sciences.* Albany, NY: SUNY Press.

Rogers, M. E. (1970). *An introduction to the theoretical basis of nursing.* Philadelphia: F. A. Davis.

Rogers, M. E. (1986). Science of unitary human beings. In V. Malinski (Ed.), *Explorations on Martha Rogers' science of unitary human beings* (pp. 3–8). Norwalk, CT: Appleton-Century-Crofts.

Rogers, M. E. (1990). Nursing: Science of unitary, irreducible, human beings: Updated 1990. In E. Barrett (Ed.), *Visions of Rogers' science-based nursing* (pp. 5–11). New York: National League for Nursing.

Smith, M. (1999). Caring and science of unitary human beings. *Advances in Nursing Science, 21,* 14–28.

Smith, M. (2004). *Transtheoretical discourse on the unitary worldview.* Keynote address at the ninth Martha E. Rogers Conference, New York University, New York.

Tyler, R. (1949). *Basic principles of curriculum and instruction.* Chicago: University of Chicago Press.

Watson, J. (1999). *Postmodern nursing and beyond.* Edinburgh, UK: Churchill Livingstone.

Watson, J. (2005). *Caring science as sacred science.* Philadelphia: F. A. Davis.

Watson, J., & Smith, M. (2002). Caring science and the science of unitary human beings: A trans-theoretical discourse for nursing knowledge development. *Journal of Advanced Nursing, 37*(5), 452–461.

11

Caring in Advance Practice Education: A New View of the Future

MARY ENZMAN HINES, RN, PhD, CNS, CPNP, AHN-BC

It has been predicted that our greatest advances in the next decade will not come from technology but from our deeper understanding of what it means to be a human, spiritual being.
—*Aburdene, 2007*

DESCRIPTION AND BACKGROUND/ OVERVIEW OF PROGRAM

Curriculum for Advance Nursing Practice

THE DOCTORATE OF NURSING PRACTICE (DNP) is a new approach to doctoral education for clinical practice. In 2006, the American Association of Critical Care Nurses (AACN) provided guidance for the development of the DNP and published eight essentials that provided a focus for the degree and the educational institutions that chose to incorporate the new degree program within schools and colleges of nursing. This provided guidance for the creation of doctoral programs for advance practice. In our college, the philosophy for the curriculum was based on a caring model, integrating Carper's (1978) patterns of knowing, White's (1995) sociopolitical knowing and Munhall's (1993) unknowing, Watson's (1988, 2005, 2008) concepts of caring and transpersonal healing, and Newman's (2008) concepts of nursing. This model was expanded to include the unitary transformative paradigm embracing reflective practice (Johns, 2004, 2009) and unitary appreciative inquiry (Cowling, 1993, 2008; Cowling & Repede, 2010) as the conceptual framework for the DNP program. Faculty and students are grounded in the belief that nursing is caring in the human health experience (Newman, Sime, & Corcoran-Perry 1991; Newman, Smith, Pharris, & Jones 2008). The curriculum for all three programs at the college (Baccalaureate, Masters, DNP) is grounded in a holistic philosophy with an understanding of nursing as a practice discipline with caring as its core. "To study nursing is to study caring, to grow in an understanding of self and other as caring person, and to be committed to the development of caring knowledge and the value of caring to the health and wholeness of persons nursed" (Boykin & Schoenhofer, 2001, pp. 55–60). In our graduate program, six major guides underpin the program: (1) nursing is a practice discipline, (2) nursing knowledge comes from multiple patterns of knowing, (3) nursing is a profession with caring at its core, (4) person/client/patient are whole beings that are interconnected with their environment and others through caring, (5) nurses are informed and experience caring in their interactions with self and other, and (6) reflective practice transforms the experiences and knowledge gained in practice to envision future practice.

In the DNP program, students begin their program of study with a theory course titled, Advanced Clinical and Holistic Health Care (Exhibit 11.1).

Reflective Practice as Framework for Caring Curriculum

Reflective practice has served as a philosophical-pedagogical underpinning to enable learning of caring within the DNP. According to Johns (2004, 2009), reflection is learning through our everyday experiences and realizing a vision for desirable practice. Johns (2009) outlines the reflective process with a variety of pedagogical guides, moving a nurse from doing reflection to experiencing reflection as a way of being (Table 11.1). Additionally, reflection is "a critical and reflexive process of self-inquiry and transformation of being and becoming the practitioner you desire to be ... reflection is always purposeful, moving towards a more reflective, effective and satisfactory life ... a special quality of being ... an awareness of self within the moment, having a clear mind so as to open to the possibility of that moment" (Johns, 2009, p. 3–4). The reflective process guides the nurse to a stillness of inner space where the mind can contemplate cognitively and affectively reveal the essence of wholeness within

COURSE TITLE: *NURS 701:* Advanced Clinical and Holistic Health Care

COURSE DESCRIPTION: Explores theoretical and philosophic foundations of reflective practice within human caring in a unitary transformative paradigm. Provides overview of principles of reflective practice, advanced practice skills, holistic therapies, and care delivery models. Advanced decision making for assessing populations/communities and clinical documentation/protocol/ clinical directives will be discussed.

OBJECTIVES

1. Articulate the interrelationships among reflective practice, research, and theory.
2. Compare and contrast philosophical traditions that influence the development of cocreative patient care.
3. Explore issues related to diagnostic testing and patient centered care.
4. Critique published research and clinical practice protocols for advanced clinical procedures.
5. Develop skills to utilize data-based development and management programs for advanced care.
6. Utilize national databases and protocols for identifications of problems and solutions within specific patient populations.
7. Develop skills to enhance expertise in advanced clinical practice.
8. Explore the concepts within advanced decision making as they apply to your new DNP role.
9. Integrate holistic philosophy and principles of practice into your emerging roles as a DNP.
10. Select appropriate tool and guides to enhance clinical documentation and protocol/clinical directives.

EXHIBIT 11.1   Advanced clinical and holistic health-care exemplar course description and objectives.

an experience (Wagner, 2008). According to Johns (2009, p. 17), reflection is "empowering and enables the practitioner to act on insight towards realizing desirable practice." Johns (2009) outlines the reflective process with a variety of pedagogical guides, moving a nurse from doing reflection to experiencing reflection as a way of being (Table 11.1)."

Practice, even in its hardest times and with all its commitments, provides the nurse a glimmer of a caring potential (Johns, 2009).

TABLE 11.1   Reflective Practice Pedagogical Guide

		Doing Reflection
Reflection on-experience	Reflecting on a situation or experience after the event with the intention of gaining insights that may inform my future practice in positive way	
Reflection in-action	Pausing within a particular situation or experience in order to make sense of and reframe the situation in order to proceed towards desired outcomes	
The internal supervisor	Dialoguing with self while in conversation with another in order to make sense	
Reflection within-the-moment	Being aware of the way I am thinking, feeling, and responding within the unfolding moment whilst holding the intent to realize my vision. It involves dialoguing with self to ensure I am interpreting and responding congruently to whatever is unfolding and having mental acuity to change my ideas rather than being fixed to certain ideas	
Mindfulness	Seeing things for what they really are without distortion, while holding the intention of realizing desirable practice	Reflection as a way of being

From: Johns, C. (2009). *Becoming a reflective practitioner* (3rd ed., p. 10). Ames, IA: Wiley-Blackwell.

Reflective practice assists the nurse in capturing the essence of caring in practice and relationships. The realization of caring within practice can be profoundly satisfying and sustaining, nourishing the commitment and purpose for practice. As van Manen (1990) captured, "retrieving or recalling the essence of caring is not a simple matter of simple etymological analysis or explication of the usage of the word. Rather, it is the construction of a way of life to live the language of our lives more deeply, to become more truly who we are when we refer to ourselves [as nurses]" (p. 58).

Within the holistic, caring curriculum model, faculty and students acknowledge that the transpersonal healing experience is the most desirable outcome for nursing/patient care (Figure 11.1).

This transpersonal healing experience occurs when the advance practice nurse (APN) and the patient exchange energy, healing, and thought in such a way that the patient has a sense of greater harmony, peace, and health; and a capacity for self-healing. The meaning of this experience is interpreted by both participants, and each has a subjective sense that she/he has experienced profound change. The APN

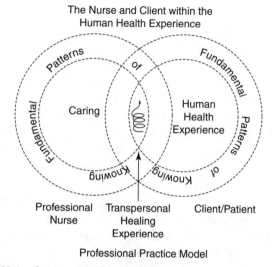

FIGURE 11.1 Conceptual model of nursing program, University of Colorado, Colorado Springs.

and the individual bring the potential of healing to each encounter, which influences the outcome of care. Both the APN and the patient have a core of experience that is influenced by patterns of knowing.

The APN's patterns of knowing are filtered through the lens of specialized nursing knowledge derived from education, research, and practice. Engaging various patterns of knowing, individuals use empirical knowledge to realize the measurable, observable aspects of life and statements of fact or descriptions of events, ethical knowledge is formulated from values and beliefs that guide and direct how nurses conduct their practice, aesthetic knowing is an appreciation, valuing and openness to wholeness and is dependent on a cultural context and background, a calling forth of the creative resources that transform experience into what is possible, sociopolitical knowing informs and allows the nurse to interact as a citizen, personal knowing informs the nurse about the inner experience of becoming a whole, aware, and genuine self and through knowing self is able to know others. Unknowing allows the person(s) to come from a place of questioning and quest to know where all things are possible. All of these patterns of knowing—empirical, ethical, aesthetic, personal, sociopolitical and unknowing—interact with events and contexts that shape an individual's life journey. Health is a part of this life journey. Within this realm, the APN and the individual encounter each other.

The core of nursing is caring in the human health experience, but caring from the particular perspective of the art and science of professional nursing. This caring core defines the content, process, context, and moral imperatives of nursing. For caring to be the content, process, context, and moral imperative for nursing, caring must be integrated with all patterns of nursing knowledge.

Through nursing education and practice, the moral imperative of caring is realized; and patterns of nursing knowledge are created, developed, and integrated into nursing as an art and science, embracing a holistic philosophical base. Furthermore, nursing education provides the opportunity for people who want to embrace this art and science to be transformed into safe, effective, caring practitioners.

The APN enters into the human health experience of the other with the knowledge, skill, ability, and personal qualities of warmth, empathy, and congruence necessary to make the possibility of transpersonal healing a reality. The curriculum focuses on the development of understanding and the skill of applying each of the patterns of knowing, especially as they relate to caring behaviors, actions, and therapeutic interventions.

The call is out to APNs to imagine the possibilities for enhancing their caring practices in the 21st century. It is the responsibility of the APN to define the essence of practice through the translation of knowledge, theory, and research.

For the APN, a centering on the consciousness and intentionality of both self and patient occurs by integrating the different types of knowledge about the disease/illness or health condition. This approach aids in the development of clinical practices based on caring, healing, and wholeness. The nurse's moral commitment, intentionality, and personal use of the clinical caritas protects, enhances, and potentiates human dignity, wholeness, and healing; this encourages the patient to create (or, really, cocreate) a meaning of a disease and treatment. The call is out to APNs to imagine the possibilities for enhancing their caring practices in the 21st century.

Whole Person Learning for Personal/Professional Development/Evolution of Creative, Liberating, Emancipatory, Spirit-Filled Approaches

The curriculum of the graduate program at University of Colorado at Colorado Springs (UCCS) is offered fully online for the DNP program. This provided a challenge for faculty who were fond of the face-to-face encounters with students. Pedagogical challenges emerged as faculty tried to take teaching strategies from the classroom to the online platform. New approaches were developed that included threaded discussions, use of Web sites and webcams, media (audio, video) powerpoints with/without embedded narration, podcasting, and outside experiences that exposed students to healing modalities and application of course material to the clinical setting. A variety of strategies have been integrated into courses that facilitate the interaction of faculty and students in the discovery of caring encounters within practice, self-knowing, and patient encounters. Consistent with the philosophical beliefs of the program, students explore their roles of scientist, artist, carer, ethicist, and global citizen that contribute to the health and well-being of individuals, communities, and diverse populations (vulnerable, rural, urban, and culturally diverse). A teaching-learning environment is facilitated with a caring, respectful, and safe environment that is developed at the beginning and throughout the course. Teaching processes of faculty have adopted a learner-centered approach rather than a teacher-centered approach. Students and faculty cocreate the learning environment and share their expertise in the threaded discussion on varied topics. Learning is focused on whole brain learning and unfolds in unique patterns for individual students. Faculty provide the context for students to acquire skills in critical analysis, formal writing, synthesis knowledge, and computer and oral skills of discussion and debate.

Creative Teaching-Learning Activities

To facilitate online learning, I developed an approach to online discussion, naming this approach SOPHIA (Speak Out, Play Havoc, Imagine Alternatives). This format provides a framing/summary for students to actively participate in an online threaded discussion. The idea of the SOPHIA was inspired by Chinn and Wheeler's (1995, p. 33) *Peace and Power* and was adapted for use as an online format for group discussion. Using the SOPHIA, the faculty provides an overview of the unit with thought questions. Students are assigned to the roles of framer and summarizer who work together as a team to start and maintain the discussion platform in the online unit. Peers are asked to provide scholarly dialogue with references to enhance the ongoing discussion about topics within the course (see Table 11.2 for an exemplar of the SOPHIA in a course). An additional approach to online threaded discussions is the Reflective Cases format for student posting and critique of a reflective narrative in practice. Two students are partnered and each student is asked to post a reflective case study on an encounter in practice related to the topic offered in unit of study. Each student uses one of three MSR formats posed by Johns (2009) (Tables 11.3, 11.4 and 11.5) for critiquing the case and then posts the response to the narrative. Each of these formats for threaded discussion asks students to direct the discussion, and the course faculty serves as guide to other resources. Additionally, students are encouraged to post resources in the webliography section (an online annotated bibliography site) of the course to enhance peer knowledge about the issues posted in the course.

Table 11.2 SOPHIA Discussion Format Exemplar

Framer (SC)

Beginnings are full of energy: anticipation, anxiety, tentativeness, even fear. All these emotions create feelings or energy in each of us.

Energy therapy is learning how to focus and move with our energy to achieve our desires. Have we learned to focus our energy (intent) and move calmly forward or are we unfocussed and showering our energy everywhere? Do we feel like our energy is stuck or not moving? Can we begin to use our energy to heal others in our roles as nurses and caregivers?

As we **begin** this module, let's take our own individual energy inventory:

As I **"begin"** my inventory, take a moment to center myself, placing my feet on the ground, taking a deep, cleansing breath. The dog also sighs. I am once again at the computer late at night. I remember this ritual of deep breathing. I used it all the time when the disaster radio went off in the ED late in my twelve hour shift.

My mind wanders to the assignments posted on the syllabi, anxiety bubbles up and I am thinking perhaps a double martini would be a better choice. Ah already off course and I am only 5 minutes into the framing! My energy is scattered. I do have lots to learn.

To **begin** the journey as holistic nurses, we have needed to connect with those transformational events that helped inform our practice. We have come to know ourselves better through the DNP course work. Our more "authentic self" is now ready to be shared with co-workers, patients and families.

This module **begins** by exploring *Healing Energy, Caring and Rituals*. We are asked to examine our caring rituals as holistic nurses. We are **beginning** to learn how to tap into the universal energy and use it to transform and heal.

We can learn to create a sacred space for healing ourselves and our patients. We already know how to create a "sacred space" for learning. We are using our sacred learning rituals of framing and summarizing. Once again we have come together in another **beginning**.

So as we **begin** this module, how are your energy levels? Are you taping into the universal energy to rejuvenate and cultivate your work? Are you using expressions of sacred rituals in your practice such as prayer, energy, humor and music?

Respondent (EG)

I was reflecting on SC's opening and pulled out Davis's book where she speaks about how to be your body psychic. She posits that "you can focus on being an empath (the ability to physically feel what others are feeling in various parts of the body) or you can focus on the abilities to sense others' body energy" (Davis, 2007, p. 6). So how often do we focus on our own body; or do we? I would posit that we do not focus often enough (even those trained)! We do not focus nearly enough time on our own life and well-being.

I know my own frailties of non focus include: (children (4), grandchildren (7), career, school. etc . . . Where am I (me) in this mix. . .? AND why do I feel guilty in wanting time for **SELF**!

Well, I try to center and focus on each opportunity and encounter. I meditate on my hour long drive to the university. I keep my office lit by lamps (not the overhead fluorescents) a student walked right by my office today and came back and said . . . "Mrs G . . . your office is never this bright . . . it is always peaceful". How nice is that comment!! I continue to search myself for ways to spend time with myself!

Reference:

Davis, N. (2007). *Be a body psychic: A simple way to read the body intuitively*. New York: Stellar Wellness Services.

Peer Response (JJ)

SC: You ask how is our energy level. This week has not been a very high energy week for me. I have patients that seemed more needful and I want to give, I have felt fragmented and somewhat guilty about time away from family. This has seemed a week of too many "have to's" and not enough of reminding myself I have choices and there are really no "have to's" with myself, my family, my co-workers or my patients. This has been a week that I have considered what is holistic and realize that though we are beginning this module that my beginning of learning about holism started several years ago when I realized that I was not balanced much less able to provide care to the patients that I was caring for. I find that I am not very good at maintaining sacred space for myself though I try to create it for my patients. I have much to learn still about balancing. This week I have used a ritual to center that in the past I have not considered a ritual- it is very simple, before I go into a room with a patient I will tap knuckles with my medical assistant- this seems to calm me and allows me to move forward. She finds it amusing but I find it calming. Thank you for the beginning. JJ

Table 11.3   The Model for Structured Reflection

Reflective Cues for Peer Critique

- Bring the mindful home
- Focus on a description of an experience that seems significant in some way
- What issues are significant to pay attention to?
- How do I interpret the way people are feeling and why they felt that way?
- How was I feeling and what made me feel that way?
- What was I trying to achieve and did I respond effectively? (aesthetic)
- What were the consequences of my actions on the patient, others, myself?
- What factors influence the way I was/am feeling, thinking and responding to the situation? (personal)
- What knowledge did or might have informed me? (empirical)
- To what extent did I act for the best and in tune with my values? (ethical)
- How does the situation connect with previous experiences? (personal)
- How might I reframe the situation and respond more effectively given this situation again? (reflexivity)
- What would be the consequences of alternative actions for the patient, others, myself?
- What factors might constrain me responding in a new ways?
- How do I NOW feel about this experience?
- Am I more able to support myself and others better as a consequence?
- What insights have I gained?
- Am I more able to realize desirable practice? (framing perspective)

From: Johns, C. (2009). *Becoming a reflective practitioner* (3rd ed., p. 51). Ames, IA: Wiley-Blackwell.

Table 11.4   Ethical Mapping

Patient/family's perspective /other patients	Who had authority to make the decision/act within the situation	The doctor's perspective
If there is conflict of perspectives/values, How might these be resolved	**The situation/dilemma**	What ethical principles inform the situation? (Beneficence, malevolence, autonomy, utilitarianism, duty and virtue, moral imperative)
The nurse's perspective	Consider the power relationships/factors that determined the way the decision/action was actually taken	The organization's perspective

From: Johns, C. (2009). *Becoming a reflective practitioner* (3rd ed., p. 77). Ames, IA: Wiley-Blackwell.

Table 11.5   Framing Perspectives Reflection

Philosophical framing How has this experience enabled Me to confront and clarify my beliefs and values that constitute desirable practice	Role framing How was this experience Enabled me to clarify my role Boundaries and authority Within my role, and my power relationships with others?	Theoretical framing/ mapping How has the experience enabled me to draw on extant theory and research in order to help me make sense of my knowing in practice, and to juxtapose and assimilate theory/ research findings with personal knowing
Developmental framing How has this experience enabled me to frame becoming a more effective practitioner within valid and appropriate theoretical frameworks/learning outcomes?	**Insights**	Reality perspective framing How has the experience enabled me to under- stand the barrier of reality whilst helping me to become empowered to act in more congruent ways?
Parallel process framing How has this experience enabled me to make connections between learning processes within my supervision process and my clinical practice?	Temporal framing How has this experience enabled me to draw patterns with past experiences while anticipating how I might respond in similar situations in new ways?	Problem framing How has this experience enabled me to focus problem identification and resolution within the experience?

From: Johns, C. (2009). *Becoming a reflective practitioner* (3rd ed., p. 78). Ames, IA: Wiley-Blackwell.

Use of Arts, Humanities, Healing Models for Learning Environment

Within the DNP program is the holistic cognate consisting of three courses that integrate the caring essence of human interaction (NURS 643 Psychobiology of Healing, NURS 647 Therapies of Energy Therapy, and NURS 648 Therapies of Imagination). In these courses is an aesthetic assignment that allows the student to investigate some aspect of the course and integrate this concept into an aesthetic expression.

A View of Caring within Advanced Practice

The stagnant view of the nurse practitioner as a "junior doctor" or physician-extender devalues the possibilities for caring to emerge for the APN in each patient encounter. Rather, an encounter between nurse practitioner and patient holds the possibility for discovering new ways of caring. Integrating caring strategies, with APN's setting an example if you will, improves the overall health for individuals, families, and communities. I pose that practices guided by a caring, humanistic philosophy hold great promise for the emerging practice models for nurse practitioners in the 21st century.

POSTSCRIPT

Critique of Program and Future Directions

My own participation in the development of a caring curriculum for doctorally prepared APNs has been thoughtful and purposeful. My time as an educator has been spent revealing nursing as a caring, healing profession. As Roach (2002) captures, caring education is for life and living, for the development of the whole person, for the formation of persons for the professions who embrace wholeness and caring as a way of life. Participating in a caring curriculum has helped me realize the depth of caring and how caring informs my interactions with those who are experiencing suffering, joy, hope, love, compassion within the human health experience. My focus for both practice and education has been on the individual's human health experience and how to realize this experience through a lens of caring. I am continually challenged to find ways to reveal these ideas to my colleagues and students.

This program is a beginning for APNs who are seeking to be challenged to see their practice in a new way. Early challenges have been experienced for both students and faculty who prior to this program had not experienced patient encounters informed by caring. Faculty educated in the traditional natural sciences approach continue to experience the challenge of this new way of experiencing humanness and health experiences that are mutually recognized and informed.

Viewing students as cocreators of knowledge has also challenged faculty who come from a lecture-based approach. The DNP program has provided an important transformational experience for all involved. The next challenge is to expand the curriculum to a BSN to DNP program.

REFERENCES

Boykin, A., & Schoenhofer, S. (2001). *Nursing as caring: A model for transforming practice*. Sudbury, MA: Jones & Bartlett.

Carper, B. (1978). Fundamental patterns of knowing in nursing. *Advances in Nursing Science, 1*(1), 13–23.

Chinn, P., & Wheeler, C. (1995). *Peace and power* (4th ed.). New York: National League of Nursing.

Cowling, W. R. (1993). Unitary knowing in practice. *Nursing Science Quarterly, 6*, 201–207.

Cowling, W. R. (2008). An essay on women, despair, and healing. *Advances in Nursing Science, 31*(3), 249–258.

Cowling, W. R., & Repede, E. (2010). Unitary appreciative inquiry evolution and refinement. *Advances in Nursing Science, 33*(1), 64–77.

Johns, C. (2004). *Becoming a reflective practitioner* (2nd ed.). Malden, MA: Blackwell Publishing.

Johns, C. (2009). *Becoming a reflective practitioner* (3rd ed.). Ames, IA: Wiley Blackwell.

Munhall, P. (1993). "Unknowing": Toward another pattern of knowing in nursing. *Nursing Outlook, 41*, 125–132.

Newman, M. (2008). *Transforming presence: The difference that nursing makes.* Philadelphia: FA Davis.

Newman, M., Sime, A., & Corcoran-Perry, S. (1991). The focus of the discipline of nursing. *Advances in Nursing Science, 14*(1), 1–6.

Newman, M., Smith, M., Pharris, M., & Jones, D. (2008). The focus of the discipline revisited. *Advances in Nursing Science, 31*(1), E16–E27.

Roach, S. (2002). *Caring, the human mode of being. A blueprint for health professionals*. Ottawa, ON: CHA Press.

van Manen, M. (1990). *Researching lived experience*. New York: The State University of New York.

Wagner, L. (2008). Caring scholar response to: Uncovering meaning through the aesthetic turn: A pedagogy of caring. *International Journal of Human Caring, 12*(2), 24–28.

Watson, J. (1988). *Nursing: Human science and human care: A theory of nursing.* New York: National League for Nursing.

Watson, J. (2005). *Caring science as sacred science*. Philadelphia: FA Davis Company.

Watson, J. (2008). *Nursing the philosophy and science of caring* (Rev. ed.). Boulder, CO: University Press.

White, J. (1995). Patterns of knowing: Review, critique, and update. *Advances in Nursing Science, 17*(4), 73–86.

12
Introduction to Caring as a Pedagogical Approach to Nursing Education

MARY ROCKWOOD LANE, PhD, RN, FAAN
MICHAEL SAMUELS, MD

T HIS CHAPTER WILL DESCRIBE COURSES that are currently taught at the College of Nursing at the University of Florida (UF) and at San Francisco State University, Holistic Studies. The two courses were developed by the authors together and have similar syllabuses. Both courses are unique interdisciplinary courses, Creativity and Spirituality in Healthcare. The Center for Spirituality and Health, which funds the UF course, has also supported several similar courses at UF in a variety of colleges. The San Francisco State University course is supported by the University and is part of their holistic health major for nurses, psychologists, and heath majors. These courses offer students an opportunity to experience their own personal spiritual journey and to explore ways in which spirituality might be integrated with their academic and career paths. In Creativity and Spirituality in Healthcare, nursing students are provided with hands-on experiences with music, dance, writing, journaling, and guided imagery. They are then encouraged to contemplate and reflect on what these experiences mean to them and what they might mean to different patient populations for whom they will care. The theory of human caring provides the philosophical and theoretical framework upon which this course was developed. This chapter will describe how the core caritas practices are foundational for the teaching and learning experience.

OVERVIEW OF PROGRAM:
PHILOSOPHICAL-THEORETICAL INFLUENCES

Jean Watson's theory of human caring is based upon the belief that the learning and teaching experience is a caring encounter. Watson's 10 core *caritas*—Latin word meaning "to cherish, to appreciate, to give special attention, if not loving, attention to" embrace the belief that trust and faith in human expression and self-actualization is the focus of the educational process. The approach of this course calls for the encouragement of contemplation and self-reflection as well as the encouragement of illumination of the human spirit. The teaching and caring process results in *caring encounters* (Watson, 1979), which are congruent with facilitation of students' engagement and emancipation.

Creativity and Spirituality in Healthcare has a scholarly component that includes: a project proposal, reading integrations, personal creative journals, and a final paper. The most significant part of the students' grades (besides attendance and participating in class) is their semester-long project and presentation that has both a personal and professional component. This project gives the students an opportunity to experience art as way of healing, as something in their own life, as well as integrating creative interventions into their chosen profession. The graduate student's final 10-page APA formatted paper must be researched and include at least seven scholarly articles relevant to the course project. Students are required to be specific in how they will weave this course material into their future jobs, clinical, etc. The project is the opportunity for the student to create a transpersonal caring experience. There are two text books required, as well as a third required text of their choice. Having this choice allows students leeway to address their own unique needs, styles, and preferences. At the beginning of the course, students are given an opportunity to meet with the faculty member for a one-on-one appointment that is geared toward student exploration of the course project and processes/activities. This is an opportunity for the faculty to bond with students and ask questions to facilitate reflection and contemplation. The following questions are indicative of this encounter:

If you could do anything you want with your life, and there were no obstacles, what is it that you would do?

- What are you most passionate about?
- Tell me about the most creative time in your life.

- Share with me your dreams and aspirations for your career, for your personal life.
- What are some of the barriers that keep you from being who you want to be, which are holding you back?
- Tell me about yourself.
- Share a life story, who you are.
- What are your hopes and desires?

Growing human consciousness that all human experience is constantly unfolding, infinitely creative, and profoundly healing, is the foundational premise of this course.

The authors highlight in their book, *Spirit-body Healing* (2000), the healing power intrinsic in the process of exploring the spirit mind-body connection. Based on the author's phenomenological hermeneutic study of creating art as a way of healing, the author proposes there is a transpersonal shift possible in the engagement of the creative process, which results in a deepening of spiritual expression and connection. This course uses creative, visionary, and spiritual practices to deepen students' journey of self-exploration and self-discovery. The entire course is an ongoing invitation for students to get in touch with their own spiritual essence and a higher power that has meaning for them. The students' journeys, themselves, create a place of healing, beauty, and grace within the ordinary setting of academia. The authors, a nurse and physician, believe it is essential for nurses to explore the authentic human experience of what it means to be a nurse.

COURSE DEVELOPMENT AND CONTENT

Creativity and Spirituality in Healthcare at UF was developed by the authors and submitted to the general College of Nursing (CON) faculty for approval to be added to the curriculum. The curriculum is reviewed by the entire faculty in the process of shared government. The course's content was perceived by the general faculty as meaningful and significant, yet the high demand of the required curriculum makes it difficult for nursing students to take electives. Since this course is not standardized in content, nor is it tested on the nursing licensure board, the content is not required. Despite this, many students have taken the course, and their feedback and evaluations have been excellent in the 5 years the course has been offered. Nursing students have also requested that this material and experience be integrated with their regular curriculum. Currently, the course remains an elective. At San Francisco State University, the course was approved by the chairman of Holistic Health as part the major and is an elective that fulfills all major requirements.

Caritas in Practice for Creation of Classroom Culture and Structure

The 10 caritas processes proposed by Watson (1979) are the foundation for creating the classroom culture and structure. In the semester sequence, the intention is to facilitate creative emergence and embracing infinite possibility, a foundational of caritas science. The classroom is a dynamic flow encompassing the appreciation of each student's individual contribution and honoring each student's subjective life journey. The caritas processes are introduced in the initial orientation to facilitate a caring and safe classroom culture.

1. *Practice Loving Kindness*

The practice of loving kindness and the process involved in authentic presence is fully subscribed in the communication dynamics of each class. For example, in the initial faculty-student meeting, each student is encouraged to experience being nurtured and to express and incorporate his or her own spiritual beliefs and practices as part of the project. The faculty demonstrates tolerance and acceptance, allowing freedom of expression, and honoring where each student is right now in their life. In the class atmosphere, there is an embracement of joy, laughter, and tears. There is an acknowledgement of the inner critic that so many of us have inside, and there is an invitation for the inner critic to wait outside the classroom doors. The students are asked to be kind and noncritical of themselves and their art. It's about process not about the outcome. The students are honored and create the flow of the manifestation of the class, which allows the students to have space. There is a fluidity and tolerance and acceptance of what is actually happening. There is an appreciation of the humanness and a tenderness in the interaction between students. The class is defined for the students as a caring community where each student is to be honored and cared for in a loving way intentionally in each encounter.

2. Instill Faith and Hope

Our classroom has the qualities of freedom, safety, trust, and collaborative expression. Students are encouraged to personally express themselves, with the witness and collaboration of others. When we create sacred space, we are intentionally shifting the environment from a traditional classroom environment into a community of harmony and balance. This is done with intention. Sacred space allows for deep listening, trusting, and faith and for the spiritual expression of each student to be honored and visible. When we create sacred space in the room, in essence we are creating sacred space both within the body and outside of the body. One technique we use to facilitate this is experiential centering and focusing activities. Faith and hope are instilled and reinforced by telling stories of how art heals and encouraging students to realize that art will heal them and their patients.

3. Nurture Individual Spiritual Beliefs and Practices

We create the sacred space that allows for a visionary and nonordinary reality to manifest. The space is pregnant with power and personal meaning. We create rituals that allow students to become connected to their own experience and what they bring to the class. Each student is invited to bring a sacred object into the physical space and share how this object is meaningful to them. In that way, each individual in the community creates an art piece in the center of the room that is a circle, places their object into a sacred circle, and integrates and interweaves diversity. They are actually placing themselves into the circle and weaving their stories together with their sacred objects. Each sacred object represents and symbolizes something deeply meaningful to each person. This may be expressed in words or just in the gift of the object. Each object is the student's own, and is deeply tied to personal meaning. The sacred space creates an altar, a place to place an object of beauty. The objects may vary from a pinecone, to a cross, to a picture of a beloved, a feather, a rock, a piece of jewelry. It depends what that person wants to contribute in that moment. The sacred space is nondenominational, does not exclude any religion, and invites everyone to participate.

Each student signs up to facilitate either an "opening" or a "closing" activity. This gives the student an opportunity to experience their own leadership of a creative/healing process. The opening shifts the space, bringing in the collaborative, collective spirit, and the closing gives a sense of completeness to the time we had been experiencing together, making a smooth transition. Some examples of these various activities are guided imagery, meditation, writing letters to loved ones, writing poetry, hand massages, yoga, stretching, sharing a significant prayer, tai chi, singing a song, playing music, leading a dance with everyone blindfolded, etc.

4. Developing Trusting–Helping Relationships

In each successive classroom meeting, the entire class contributes to developing a safe environment that supports helpful and trusting relationships between faculty and students and students and students. The checking in at the beginning of class, allows each student to share what is going on in their life and in their work. Confidentiality is important. We ask students to create a commitment that honors every student's story. The sharing is confined to the classroom, which allows students to know they are safe in their vulnerabilities if and when they choose to share. During the course, sometimes emotional stories come up. If someone cries and shares a painful story, one of the ways we handle profound emotional sharing is to honor it with a moment of pause and silence, allowing students to hold the emotional expression. Nurses need this type of experience to overcome fear or discomfort with patients needing to express this type of emotional pain. We allow it to be expressed, pause, and experience the silence in holding their story. In the beginning of the course, students are given free counseling resources in case students want to pursue counseling. This course is not a substitute for group or individual counseling, but students are encouraged to realize that they will be loved and helped when they express emotion.

5. Promote and Accept Expressions of Positive and Negative Feelings

There is integrity and wholeness in the creative expression. A painting can hold the despair of a painful experience. In the painting itself, the despair is held, acknowledged, and honored. There is a witness, and in the witnessing, that expression can be complete.

Inherent in exploring different and various creative activities, we promote and accept the expression of both positive and negative feelings. For example, students are invited to share their joys as well as their struggles as part of the class. As part of the creative process these expressions and feelings are expressed in poetry, art, music, songwriting, even dance. In students' journals, their truth is encouraged, and there are oftentimes dark and painful expressions and processing. In their reading integrations, we encourage them to critically examine and integrate the readings, and to share their personal opinions of anything they agree or disagree with or would change about how the readings apply to their understanding. One of the things this class does by integrating creative modalities is that it really opens up deep expressions of both negative and positive feelings. What manifests are incredibly exquisite art forms. These art forms contain profound and deeply felt expressions of sadness, pain, anger, hurt, grief, anxiety, fear, love, joy, appreciation, acceptance, self-awareness, etc. The images demonstrate the emotions almost more explicitly than words. What is so powerful about the manifestation of art with human expression, is that it creates something tangible emerging from the intangible depths of their humanness. The power of creative expression is the ability of the artist to reach into the dark depths of themselves, into the darkness and pain, and allow the expression of these very intense and palpable feelings. They come from the darkness within, and you bring them forth into the light. When we create art with this depth of expression, we have the ability to witness ourselves. There becomes an ability to be detached from ourselves, enough to embrace ourselves with compassion. The art gives us an opportunity to accept, embrace, and forgive ourselves, and fall in love with the beauty that we are capable of creating. Even in our sadness and fear . . . there is beauty in the ugliness when the ugliness is the truth. The truth reflects what is in each and everyone of us. It's simply a reflection of the truth of our own humanity. The course is unusual in that there are moments of deep emotional expression and revelation. Students often cry, hug each other, and become deeply connected in community with new friendships created.

6. Creative Use of Self in All Ways of Knowing, Being, and Doing

We encourage students to get connected to remembering when they were young and loved making art, when there was no inner critic. The following are examples of prompts we use to help students get in touch with their inner artist, free from self-consciousness and criticism, to experience patients in a new way and make creative connections between what they imagine (or have witnessed) and their nursing role(s).

See Beauty. How do we look at our practice as nurse-artists? It is simple: we can begin to cultivate a way of seeing from the eyes of an artist. We can learn to see beauty in the faces of people for whom we care. To see the beauty of lips, eyes—to cultivate a way of seeing that is always sensitive to the human in front of us—the tear that flows down a cheek, the hand that trembling, reaches out as we walk around the bed. Notice and experience these encounters of incredible beauty. Pause and reflect. Cultivate a way of being in the moment with the patient more deeply, more fully.

Use Voice. We can cultivate the artist's use of vibration and learn to recognize the power of our own voices. Voice used as sentiment, voice as music, a soothing tone, a soft whisper of reassurance. We can use our *nursing voices* as instruments for healing. We can project our compassion, our comfort, through our voices—filling our chests with the deep vibration that connects to the center of ours and our patients' souls. When we use voice, we come from a powerful place, we speak from our center and are grounded. Voice becomes a powerful healing tool.

Move With Grace. The nurse-artist can use the body to flow in the graceful movements of **the dancer**. Move in and out of rooms with gestures of grace, rhythm, and beauty, creating symmetry and balance within the routine rhythms of daily unit activity. Moving patients, helping them get out of bed, can be like a dance. See yourself and your patients as dance partners—leading and following, practicing the moves, until the patterns are smooth and graceful. Remember, the operative word is *practice*—and this applies to *graceful* communication as well.

Healing Touch. As nurses, we cannot overestimate the power of touch, the gift of being able to touch another human in moments of pain and suffering. We can touch with softness, healing energy, and can be connected through the textures, smells, and needs of another in sacred intimacy. We can embody intimacy as a sacred connection. Touch as you yearn to comfort, care, protect. Touch to help ease pain and transmit confidence and hope. Touch is an intuitive healing intervention we all know deep inside our bodies. For some it comes naturally; for others, awareness of sacred touch can be cultivated. For starters, remember how essential it is to be hugged once in awhile or how much joy the weight of a squiggling puppy can bring to young and old alike. In particular, remember that your hands have the power to convey caring and gentleness, just as they can convey impersonal "busy-ness." Know, too, that your eyes can "touch" others. Truly, they *are* windows to your soul.

7. Unity of Being and Subjective Meaning

The classroom climate is liberating, open, and energetic. This is a humanistic value system in which the learning experience is inherently customized to each students' needs and desires. What they need from this class is what they are going to get. Emphasis is placed on the value of innovativeness, being creative, and embodying the experience of self-exploration. The experience in each student's project is really being able to tap into their own inner resources, and each student is honored as a healer and an artist by self-discovery and inner contemplation, this experience honors the wisdom of intuition, and encouraging the student to see into their own beingness and discovery of who they are.

8. The Classroom as a Healing Environment for the Physical and Spiritual Self That Respects Human Dignity

The classroom is housed in a very traditional academic university setting. However, when the student walks into the room, there is soothing music playing, there is an art cart and art supplies on the table, art is hung on the walls, beautiful fabrics cover the tables, and are accented with arrangements of flowers and food. Thus, the student experiences an immediate and significant transition, entering a sort of portal to a different time and space. The environment is noncritical, nonjudgmental. The novelty sometimes creates awkwardness and fear about trying unfamiliar activities that may not have been engaged in since childhood, or possibly never tried before. There is much gentle encouragement to experiment, to do something they may have always wanted to do but never gave themselves permission. The environment is all about embracing newness and the moment. Students typically support each other right away and are patient with each other's reluctance or hesitance. The shared experience of discomfort or self-consciousness bonds students and encourages a level of tolerance from the start. The classroom environment is created in each class session intentionally to make a new sacred space that invites healing and protects the students from what is not healing for them.

9. Basic Needs

Since this class is typically conducted in the evening during dinnertime, students sign up to share food, snacks, and drinks. This is the caritas practice where students' basic physical needs (thirst and hunger) are met. We serve hot tea with lemon—this is cleansing, healthy, and provides unique sharing. The invitation to share food is another opportunity to be creative. Food can actually be part of the art-making process, or it can simply serve to quench hunger. For some students, food can serve to help decrease stressful feelings. This class also meets the basic need of stress relief. Many students have shared that this class is something they really look forward to each week. There is a lightness and opening that really is nourishing for them. Students can step out of a stressful, rigorous, high-pressured, information-heavy, high-tech, overbusy lifestyle, and rejuvenate their energy.

10. Allow Space for Miracles to Take Place

The most wonderful caritas process is allowing the space for miracles to take place. Many of the students' projects are deeply healing and transformative, and in the presentation and sharing, there are moments that are so heart-opening and that produce so much awe and revelation, they are truly miraculous. Students are prepared for this by constantly hearing and sharing stories of miracles in art and healing. Web sites and stories of patients and artists are shared that are exemplars for miracles in healing. The openness of the class allows a natural flow where an energetic field is created where a miracle reveals itself. It can't be planned, but gives permission for a magical deeply spiritual energy to appear and be illuminated and the miracles are witnessed and seen as they are experienced. As students share, they are even astonished by their own experience of themselves. The mystery of who they are is revealed to themselves. There is such exquisite beauty in that that it is a miracle and give you goose bumps.

There is rarely repetition, there is not formula, which manifests a much more interesting experience. In the time allowed for the classroom there is a natural flow that evolves. Sharing and expressing of what would have never been able to be anticipated. Inside this creative freedom the student can evolve within themselves, as themselves within a caring community that honors and witnesses their illumination and their growth. What is truly remarkable is the unfolding of the mystery as each student's humanness is revealed in the moment. These moments are indescribable and exquisitely beautiful. They are *miraculous* moments.

Pedagogical Practices: Examples of Transformative Liberating Approaches to Teaching Learning

The class is organized like a seminar. Teachers and guest speakers (artists, poets, dancers, actresses, yoga teachers, clowns, etc.) are guides and facilitators rather than lecturers. Students are gathered in a circle seated in chairs with a desk in the center. There is no hierarchal presentation of faculty.

Creative teaching/learning activities examples:

JOURNAL WRITING

We invite students in the class to allow themselves to connect with their inner artist with daily journal writing. The journal is brought to class and students continue to journal as the class takes place. The journal is a portable studio, accessible for self-expression and self-reflection.

The Journals are a place where people can find the place of their own compassionate, wise, inner truth. The students can shamelessly discover what they are sometimes afraid to say out loud. They paint, draw, write, color, collage, decorate their journals with meaningful quotes, poems, etc. Diverse mediums are set out to allow the students to explore which art materials resonate with them. The journals are a place for students to externalize their internal confusion, clarity, pain, joy, anger, gratitude, etc. Students are amazed at what their journal pages reveal to them about their inner workings. One journal writing exercise is called Vigali's Questions. The students do a guided imagery about what is their essence, what is blocking them from connecting to their essence, and what can they do to see their essence manifest.

Music as Healing

Music engenders a sense of community throughout the semester. We invite students to bring in CDs to play as background music for each weekly class while they are amidst the creative processes. Class members are exposed to new musical possibilities as students share their musical interests with one another. One of our classes each semester has music in the foreground, where we concentrate on the therapeutic value of music.

Youtube videos can be very transformative, evocative, relaxing, empowering, etc. Songs and lyrics can bring up very relevant and deep-seeded emotional resonances. This is relevant to nurses because with modern technology, with an ipod or computer, patients can be guided from a lonely and isolated place, to feeling connected, and having their situation normalized through even just one 3-minute music video. Various artists have taken traumatic, painful situations, diseases, loss, suffering, death awareness, etc. and shown how beauty can be created from the ugliest of circumstances.

We demonstrate this in a classroom setting by playing one YouTube video at a time, in the dark, and then having a 5-minute pause after each one, where we turn the lights back on and the students respond in their journals. A packet of lyrics is distributed to the students so they can process and personalize what the messages mean to them.

There are often very strong reactions. For example, a very significant lesson happened when one of the facilitators showed a song that addressed child abuse. Showing music videos about child abuse can ignite powerful and enlightening dialogue, healing opportunities, heightened awareness, and compassion. Child abuse is one of the many harsh realities of life that nursing students may be exposed to in their hospital settings.

After presenting the prepared YouTube videos, the students get an opportunity to share their own examples of music that is healing, therapeutic, and transformative in their lives.

Dancing

Create an atmosphere of comfort, safety . . . lowering the lights . . . candles (electric if not allowed), light lamps. The students are encouraged to dance, in class exercises, breaks, and with each other. Dance facilitated movement, freeing healing energy, and group bonding. It is social for young people, they know it well and enjoy it, but they may never have used it intentionally for healing. Dance activities are taught such as one person leading another blindfolded person in a dance, to encourage trust, partnering and dancing a story of an illness and healing and dancing as healers around a person who asks to be healed. We move the tables and chairs so there is room to dance freely. Dance is present in the class and flows over to the students lives. Students often remained after class drumming and dancing when class was long over.

Visual Art Projects

Students do visual art after each guided imagery. They draw what they image to see more deeply. They draw for more than a half hour after each guided imagery and become used to using visual arts to heal and see deeper. It is an integral part of the class, students sit and draw in their journals as class takes place, it becomes natural, healing, and powerful and is often the beginning of their projects.

The story of my body: In this class we paired the students up. We laid out a long roll of paper, and one student lay down on it at a time, to be traced by their partners and that student traced the other student's outline. The next person lay on the table and they were traced. Then they used markers, crayons, collage, magazine articles, to color the figures in and make them become alive.

Collage

Students do a self-portrait collage. This was an intuitive process to find something they resonate with without thinking. It was spontaneous, and the students could share the collage, and discuss what the collage meant to them. They could talk about the metaphors within the words and images, and how that related to a deep meaningful part of who they are.

Art Cart

There are a variety of art supplies (pastels, watercolor kits, stickers, ribbons, magazines, multiple color and designed papers, glue sticks, colored markers, pencils, etc.)

Drama

In our drama/theater in health-care class, our class members participate in theater games that entail playful improvisational interactions. These games give opportunities for students to go outside their comfort zone and play. The movement and self-expression allows the nervousness to dissipate and creates an atmosphere of fun and playfulness. We intentionally have the theater class in the beginning of the semester because the laughter and liberated energy that is created from the theater games and playback can take down walls and dissolve the awkwardness that students sometimes come in with. Openness and comfort is fostered. In the theater games, students are invited to take on various emotions and roles. They can take on different emotions and characters and go beyond their persona. This class has a guest facilitator who is an artist in resident who works with patients in the hospital with her playback troupe. This focuses on listening intently to someone's personal story and then reflecting back to that person an enactment of that story. This can be profoundly validating and healing to witness the externalization of such an internal and emotional experience. In our class, one way this was demonstrated was by a student who volunteered to share her story of being depressed and overwhelmed with her life, feeling pulled in so many different directions, wearing so many different hats in her life, and not knowing how to juggle all these seemingly competing roles. A group of her classmates was assigned the role of representing the various aspects of her life that were pulling on her and competing for her attention (her own personal health, her family, her husband, graduate school, work, etc.). Each person acting out each valid part of her was talking over one another, demanding that their needs be met. In the process of this being acted out and demonstrated in such a realistic way, many students in the class related to this overwhelmed feeling, and a few students shed tears, feeling so validated and having their struggle being shown in this way. A very genuine empathy was created because so many students (and obviously patients) can relate to feeling stressed out in their own lives.

Guest Artists

There is a spontaneousness and openness to what they bring to each class. Every semester the course is taught it is never the same as it was before. The guest speakers are available for information and to be a resource to the students inside and outside the classroom. The guest speakers enjoy sharing their artistic talents, in essence give the student opportunity to explore new and innovative ways to be creative. Guest artists in art and healing also allow the students to see art and healing professionals, know other ways of teaching, and realize the art and healing field is large and has different points of view.

STRUCTURE OF CURRICULUM FRAMEWORK

The curriculum in which this course is offered is a traditional undergraduate/graduate nursing program. At UF, there is a strong focus on research, quantitative and measurement of evidence based. This course is in the college of nursing that is one of six health science colleges in a major academic state public system. At the San Francisco State University, the curriculum matches the 12-weekly model of a usual 3-credit course.

Course Description Example

NUR 4930/6930: Spirituality and Creativity in Health care

This course gives undergraduate and graduate students in nursing, art, and other disciplines an overview of the field of Spirituality, Creativity, and Health care. It will describe the history and physiology of Spirituality, Creativity in Health care, explain the use of art, writing, music, and dance to heal, provide exemplars of programs that use creativity and spirituality to heal, and demonstrate the praxis of artists healing themselves, others, and the earth. The course utilizes stories of patients and artists, and guided imagery as a way of teaching. Creative art projects provide exciting opportunities for personal growth and healing. The final art project can be any art process that heals. Students have built meditation sanctuaries in their homes for peace, written poetry for a brother who was ill, painted their inner critic and inner artist, created portfolios of healing photographs, sculptures, or painting, and created art programs in health-care settings. This course shows how art, spirituality, and healing are one. It shows how creativity and spirituality resonate the body, mind, and spirit and talks about how art is transformational to us, others, and the earth. The course discusses the future of art, spirituality, and healing and talks about how spirituality and health-care departments in universities are now helping people pray and use spiritual disciplines to heal. This course is about healing your own spirit.

Course Sequence

Initially, we go over the syllabus, provide a question and answer period, and immediately begin to establish the structure of free forum of ideas between all participants.

Example of syllabus

UNIVERSITY OF FLORIDA

COLLEGE OF NURSING
COURSE SYLLABUS
Fall 2009

COURSE NUMBER	NUR 4930—section #2861
	NGR 6930—section # 2853
COURSE TITLE	Spirituality and Creativity in Health Care
CREDITS	3
PLACEMENT	Elective
PREREQUISITES	None
COREQUISITES	None
FACULTY	

Mary Rockwood Lane, RN, PhD Clinical Associate Professor mlane@health.ufl.edu	HPNP 3210	273-6371	By appointment
Emi Lenes, Med/EdS, NCC Em00017@ufl.edu	HPNP 3210	682-9594	By appointment
DEPARTMENT CHAIR			
Maxine M. Hinze, RN, PhD hinzemm@nursing.ufl.edu	HPNP 3230	273-6394	Mon. 1–2; Tues. 1–2 or by appointment

(*continued*)

COURSE SCHEDULE

Days	Time	Room
Thursday	5:10–8:10	HPNP 3203/3203A

COURSE DESCRIPTION: This course provides an overview of spirituality and creativity in health care and extends the student's knowledge of the creative arts in human caring. It will provide an understanding of the use of visual arts, writing, music, and creative movement. Emphasis will be placed on the artistry of caring and spiritual praxis in holistic care. The focus will be self-utilization of the creative arts, guided imagery, and meditative practices.

COURSE OBJECTIVES: Upon completion of the course, the student will be able to:

1. Utilize knowledge and theory from the humanities and caring arts to provide a foundation for human caring practice.
2. Apply the creative arts process and guided imagery techniques to facilitate the human expression of a mind, body, spirit experience of wholeness.
3. Apply health-care therapeutics of the creative arts, guided imagery, and meditative practices to nursing practice.
4. Distinguish the ways in which artistic mediums are utilized to promote healing in health care.
5. Explain the steps of creativity as they facilitate a deeper understanding of spiritual health.

ATTENDANCE
Students are expected to be present for all classes, other learning experiences, and examinations. Students who have extraordinary circumstances preventing attendance should explain these circumstances to the course instructor **prior** to the scheduled class as soon as possible. Instructors will make an effort to accommodate *reasonable* requests. A grade penalty may be assigned for late assignments or make-up exams. Make-up exams may not be available in all courses.

ACCOMMODATIONS DUE TO DISABILITY
Each semester, students are responsible for requesting a memorandum from the Office for Students with Disabilities to notify faculty of their requested individual accommodations. This should be done at the start of the semester.

STUDENT HANDBOOK
Students are to refer to the College of Nursing Student Handbook for information about College of Nursing policies, honor code, and professional behavior.

(*continued*)

TOPICAL OUTLINE
1. Overview of the field of arts in medicine and spirituality in health care
2. Guided imagery and research that supports the healing physiology of spirit body healing
3. History; use of creativity and spirituality in healing through the ages
4. The health professional as the ontological artist for caring and healing
5. Visual arts in health care
6. Music in health care
7. Dance in health care
8. Poetry, journaling, and storytelling in health care
9. The creative arts as advanced nursing therapeutics
10. Community healing art
11. Application of art in spirituality in practice

TEACHING METHODS
Lecture, discussion, group work, guest lectures, art projects, audiovisual materials, demonstrations, and exercises.

LEARNING ACTIVITIES
Active participation, journaling, experiential creative processing, written papers, group processing, reading integration, project proposal, final project, presentations.

EVALUATION METHOD/COURSE GRADE CALCULATION
Class participation, written and artist journals, scholarly paper and healing art project.
(Note: specific guidelines will be included in the course materials. Student enrolled for graduate credit will have higher-level requirements specified.)
COURSE REQUIREMENTS:
Each student will:

1. Attend each class/Participate in class discussion and projects.
2. Create plan for a significant project you will be implementing.
3. Work throughout the semester on this project that explores the spiritual dimension of healing yourself and others.
4. Read assignments prior to class. Write a paper integrating the readings.
5. Create a personal journal—bring to class each week.
6. Prepare a written paper on your selected project. Students taking the course for graduate credit will require a more in-depth scholarly paper.

(*continued*)

Your grades are based on:

1. Attendance/Participation—Total points is 30 points, with each class period being worth 2 points, and a required half hour one-on-one meeting with each facilitator that is worth 1 point each meeting.
2. Project Proposal—**Due September 24.** A detailed description and timeline of your project.
3. Creativity in Healing Project—focus on own healing process and implementing a creative process with others. This project can be done individually or in pairs. Instructor approval required. Please do a project that stretches you. You will be presenting this project to the class.
4. Reading Integration—3 pages. **DUE November 5.** You may compare/contrast, critically analyze, and find a common thread throughout the readings for this class. Synthesize and justify the authors' writings and how they relate to and affect you. Include specific examples from at least 3 different readings.
5. Weekly journal entry—Please bring your updated journal to class each week, we will be working on our journals in class as well. You will be assigned a weekly journal entry. **Turned in November 19.**
6. **Your final paper is due December 3.**
   - Undergraduate Students: Write a 3–5 page paper describing your creative process and project implementation. Include 3 sources. Please illustrate your depth of understanding of the articles. See Grading Rubric on the last page of the syllabus.
   - Graduate Students: Research scholarly articles related to your project on Spirituality, Creativity, and Health care. Write a 6–8 page paper describing your creative process and project implementation. Be specific in how you will weave this course material into your future jobs, clinicals, etc. Please use APA format. Must include at least 7 sources and 3 primary sources. Please indicate the future implications of this course in your life.

GRADING SCALE

A	94–100	C	74–81*
B+	92–93	D+	72–73
B	84–91	D	64–71
C+	82–83	E	63 or below

* 74 is the minimal passing grade

(*continued*)

COURSE GRADE CALCULATIONS

Attendance/Participation	30% of total grade
Creative Healing Project/Presentation	25% of total grade
Student Journal	20% of total grade
Reading Integration	10% of total grade
Student Paper	10% of total grade
Project Proposal	5% of total grade

REQUIRED TEXTS

1. Samuels, M. and Lane, M. (2000). *Spirit Body Healing.* New York: Wiley and Sons.
2. Samuels, M. and Lane, M. (2003). *Shaman Wisdom.* New York: Wiley and Sons.
3. See List of Choices for 3rd required Book.

RECOMMENDED TEXTS

Fox, M. (2002). *Creativity.* New York: Tarcher.
Watson, J. (1999). *Postmodern Nursing and Beyond.* Edinburgh, NY: Churchill Livingstone.

WEEKLY CLASS SCHEDULE

DATE	TOPIC/ EVALUATION	ASSIGNMENTS/ READINGS	FACULTY
August 27	Introduction/ Names Color My World Project Examples	Spirit Body Healing Ch. 1–3 Journal Entry— spiritual history	M. Lane Emi Lenes
September 3	Guided Imagery, Create Sacred Space, Sharing Spiritual Experiences	Spirit Body Healing Ch. 4–6 Journal Entry	M. Lane Emi Lenes
September 10	Slideshow Healing Collage	Spirit Body Healing Ch. 7–9 Journal Entry	M. Lane Emi Lenes
September 17	Playback Theater/ Drama & Healing/Self Reflective Storytelling	Spirit Body Healing Ch. 10–11 Journal Entry	M. Lane Emi Lenes Paula Paterson

(*continued*)

DATE	TOPIC/ EVALUATION	ASSIGNMENTS/ READINGS	FACULTY
September 24	Feedback on Projects Intuitive Painting	Spirit Body Healing Ch. 12–epilogue **Project Proposal Due** Journal Entry	M. Lane Emi Lenes
October 1	Music and Healing	Shaman Wisdom Ch. 1–3 Journal Entry	M. Lane Emi Lenes
October 8	Creativity and Counseling	Grace and Grit Handout Journal Entry	Emi Lenes Ana Puig Lyn Goodwin
October 15	The Story of my Body	Shaman Wisdom Ch. 7–9 Journal Entry	M. Lane Emi Lenes
October 22	Mosaics	Shaman Wisdom Ch. 10–12 Journal Entry	M. Lane Gina Zeitlin Emi Lene
October 29	Visual Art and Healing	Shaman Wisdom Ch. 13–14 Journal Entry	Mary Lisa
November 5	Death and Dying	**Reading Integrations Due** Journal Entry	Mary Lane
November 12	Alex Grey	Journal Entry	Alex Grey
November 19	Student Presentations	**Journals Due**	You!!!
November 26	Happy Thanksgiving	No class	
December 3	Student Presentations	**Final Papers Due**	You!!!
December 10	Creating Sacred Space, Ceremony	Dinner Celebration Gathering at Mary's Home	M. Lane Emi Lenes

Approved: Academic Affairs Committee: 6/02

Faculty: 6/02

UF Curriculum:

Guided imagery

Guided imagery is foundational for allowing students to access their inner world. It is a basic tool used in cancer centers for

(*continued*)

relaxation and is useful for all nurses to be able to understand and practice. We use guided imagery extensively in the class, with guided imagery exercises for experiencing the inner artist, the inner critic, the inner healer, and experience darkness, light, and healing energy.

A living example of guided imagery

Make yourself comfortable. You can be sitting down or lying down. Loosen tight clothing, uncross your legs and arms. Close your eyes. Let your breathing slow down. Take several deep breaths. Let your abdomen rise as you breathe in, and fall as you let your deep breath out. As you breathe in and out you will become more and more relaxed. You may feel feelings of tingling, buzzing, or relaxation, if you do, let those feelings increase. You may feel heaviness or lightness, you may feel your boundaries loosening and your edges softening.

Now let yourself relax. Let your feet relax, let your legs relax. Let the feelings of relaxation spread upwards to your thighs and pelvis. Let your pelvis open and relax. Now let your abdomen relax, let your belly expand, do not hold it in anymore. Now let your chest relax, let your heartbeat and breathing take place by themselves. Let your arms relax, your hands relax. Now let your neck relax, your head, your face. Let your eyes relax, see a horizon and blackness for a moment. Let these feelings of relaxation spread throughout your body. Let your relaxation deepen. If you wish you can count your breaths and let your relaxation deepen with each breath.

In your mind's eye picture yourself healing. Let the love you feel come to you and surround you. Be in the love and compassion you are given from the universe. Now imagine you are the most compassionate person you have known, heard of, read about, or imagined. Be in your heart. Let the love you are, merge with the love within your heart. Now look at yourself with pure compassion. Look through the eyes of the compassionate one. Look through your own eyes seeing yourself in the deepest love and compassion.

Now remember your own story of great suffering or pain. Listen to your own story as you are the healer. The healer is the artist within. As you hear your own story, let your love and compassion surround like a blanket from a mother to her baby. Let the love flow into your heart as you are the compassionate one. Let the suffering emerge into a sea of pure love.

Take this image and imagine yourself as an artist in total freedom creating art: A dance, a song, or a poem. You are beautiful and spontaneous. Imagine yourself being an artist. Allow yourself to play and explore, Allow whatever images emerge . . . .

When you are ready, return to the room where you are doing the exercise. First move your feet and then move your hands. Move

(*continued*)

them around and experience the feeling of the movement. Press your feet down onto the floor, feel the grounding, feel the pressure on the bottom of your feet, feel the solidity of the earth. Feel your backside on the chair; feel your weight pressing downwards. Now open your eyes. Look around you. Stand up and stretch, move your body, feel it move. You are back, you can carry the experience of the exercise outward to your life. You will feel stronger and be able to see deeper. You will be in a healing state. Each time you do the exercise you will be more relaxed and be able to go deeper and be more deeply healed.

This class is a personal journey where the student is honored as their own healer and artist. The class provides an opportunity for the student to go deeper into their own quest of their spiritual journey.

Pedagogical Practices—Examples of Transformative Liberating Approaches to Teaching

The key role of the faculty is to facilitate and empower the student. This course is a place to capture ideas and create a plan for implementation. As time goes on, the classroom becomes an increasingly sharing, caring, and cohesive community that embraces the energies and aspirations of each student. The teaching approach is active and collaborative. The classroom is a structure for open and expansive learning. The course is about tapping into the infinite potentiality for each student. It's remarkable for the class members to witness each other in the deep depths of wandering within themselves.

Just as our external physical space can be sacred, creating sacred space within the body is ultimately what is happening as well. The class provides an opportunity to slow down, leave the rest of their concerns behind, and step into another experience.

The faculty focuses the student on settling down into their sitting posture, becoming aware of their breathing, taking slow deep breaths, allowing the body to relax and go into a mediation centering experience . . .

Our Students come from diverse departments, such as Nursing, Counselor Education, Religion, Premed, Anthropology, Fine Arts, Ceramics, Photography, etc. Being all together in the classroom, students realize that no matter what their profession is, they are part of an interdisciplinary, multifaceted community of people who are also professional in many diverse and different ways. This course deepens the experience of self-awareness also allowing the students to understand the experience of other students in a powerful way.

Each class has an outline and agenda, but this class has a fluidity and it's not rigidly planned. The last half of the class is always an experiential process—engaging in making art together.

Use of Arts, Humanities, Healing Models for Learning Environment— Examples. The project is the most important part of the class. Each student does a project to actually use art—visual arts, music, dance, word, or ceremony, to heal themselves, others, neighborhood, or the earth. The project is presented to the class in a 15-minute presentation with any visuals the student wants, for example, PowerPoint, music, dance. The presentation is an intentional healing act; the student is healed by revealing their truth. In addition, a written paper is due. Below is an excerpt of the paper turned in after the presentation. In the course at San Francisco State University, the process is emphasized, not the language of the paper or writing style. The paper below was by a student with Spanish as the first language.

This is an example of a project done by a nursing student in neonatal care unit in the class at San Francisco State University.

Art as Healing for Mommy and Baby

"I am passionately committed to helping people discover their healing power, the one that lives and breathes within each of us. My mission and focus for the project was to volunteer one day each month to dedicate to healing the mothers' bodies, mind, and spirit through the creative and therapeutic process of writing and listening to poetry. My vision is to awaken this creative and healing voice in the human spirit.

I am completely dedicated to nurturing and strengthening the mothers' capacity to connect with themselves, others, and most importantly with their babies.

I brought together mothers whose babies are in the Neonatal Intensive Care Unit. They wrote a letter or a poem to their baby and, furthermore, I took a picture of the mother, father, and their baby, and I framed the picture with the poem and gave it to them as a gift. For the project, I focused on Spanish native speakers; however, anyone was welcome to participate. I am committed to helping Spanish-speaking parents through the stressful experience of hospitalization.

One of the main reasons why I thought about doing this project is because I was a preemie baby myself, and my mother wrote me a letter when I was in the Neonatal Intensive Care Unit (NICU). In the letter, she explained her painful and difficult experience in the NICU. In addition, I was only 1 pound 13 ounces when I was born, and for that reason the doctors explained to my mother that I had a very slight chance of surviving, and if I did survive I might have some health problem in the future. My mother always had hope—she explained to me that she believed in God, and she knew in her heart that I was going to survive. She always told me "think positive—never think negative." Thanks to God, I am still here on this earth, and I truly believe that this class was a sign for me. The class reopened my eyes in a good way. Thanks to the class, I am dedicated to helping others through the creative and therapeutic process of art.

Hospitals all over the world are including art into patient care. For that reason, I am glad I did this project because now I am going to volunteer in the NICU once a month to help the parents heal their bodies, mind, and spirit through the creative and therapeutic process of writing and listening to poetry. In addition, hospitalization can be stressful—problems or concerns may arise during anyone's stay, and not being able to communicate with others can make it difficult. For that reason, I created the Art as Healing for Mommy and Baby class for the Spanish-speaking parents.

I have enhanced the NICU by making it a more transnational place. In addition, helping the parents capacity to connect with themselves, others, and most importantly with their babies, puts a smile on my face.

Many times, non-English speakers feel unwelcome in the health-care system, and one of the reasons can be because of their lack of communication. Studies show that the number one factor in receiving competent care, building effective communication with Latinos in the United States, is having a Spanish-speaking health professional. But, since relatively few providers speak Spanish, the interpersonal communication between the physicians and patients can be ineffective. Communications need to be effective because many times they are dealing with people's health.

The Art as Healing for Mommy and Baby class can be a solution to the parent's current needs. When the parents are able to communicate with me as a Latina and when they can be able to express their feeling through the process of writing or poetry, a huge difference occurs.

I want to take the extra step and help parents heal their bodies, mind, and spirit though the process of art. I want to become a hero in my mothers' eyes and a role model for everyone in my community. What makes me strong is my Latina roots and my mother. Because of her, I am where I am now. I'm glad I am using my mother's experience as a way to help other people. My determination to succeed is fueled by my passion to break down barriers that keep many Latinos from excelling. I want to prove that I have persevered against all odds and I have changed my community by making it a more transnational, and nonstressful Place.

Thanks to the Art as Healing course, I learned so many things that will help me in my future. This class enabled me to understand many particular ways to be able to heal my bodies, mind, and spirit. It made me open my eyes a little more so that I can become extra curious about life. I appreciate the faculty for giving me the opportunity to expand my education about healing. The class has made me a stronger Latina, and I'm excited to continue helping others heal their bodies, mind, and spirit because I am also healing myself."

The class could not believe how beautiful this simple elegant project was. One woman, a student in a University class, changed healthcare in a neonatal unit in a one-semester project for a course. How incredible is that?

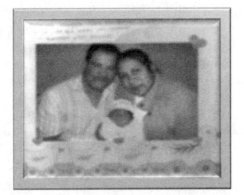

Project done by a nursing student in the neonatal intensive care unit in a class at San Francisco State University. (For a better view of photo, see http://artandhealingblog.com/lessons-from-art-as-healing-for-mommy-baby.)

Lessons From Art as Healing for Mommy Baby

In class, we talk about what we learn from the presentations. This is an example of lessons students learned from the lived experience projects:

From Art as Healing for Mommy Baby the student learned the following:

> *Passionate commitment*
> *Cross cultural awareness*
> *Mission focus dedication.*
> *Vision process emerged simple and clear*
> *Past history informed her deeply inside*
> *Based in research*
> *she became a hero and model for all*
> *Determination to succeed fueled by passion*
> *Change community, heal community*
> *Found who she was healed herself*

CONCLUSION

We want to enable the nursing students to reconnect to their own humanness, explore their own inner sense of being and their own inner world, at the same time honoring their academic and scholarly pursuits in their variety of disciplines This course is an opportunity for students to return to themselves and remember why they went into nursing in the first place. This course is an opportunity for students to return to lost parts of themselves. Many students have dreams that have been buried, disowned, or let go of, because of the academic rigor they are immersed in. When the student has gone into an academic program, they experience intense professional socialization. This course gives the student a personal opportunity to attend to obstacles that prevent them from being able to be fully present in their career decisions. One of our intentions is tapping into the students' ability to be in love with what they do academically and professionally. We ask the student provocative questions about what it is that they are going to dedicate the rest of their life to. We allow the student to have a glimpse of looking inside themselves and see deeper into the mystery of who they are. The students can go to a place where they discover and reconnect to what they are most passionate about relating to their lives' work. This opportunity allows the student to experience a shift in their reality and become more conscious of what they are going to contribute to the role of their professional life. The students then begin to remember who they are and what they bring to their profession.

This course is an opportunity for the student to contemplate who they are, what does it mean to be in this professional role, and who they are as a human being doing it. The most important thing that people bring to their career is how they authentically and uniquely are. This course calls them to go back inside and explore why they made the choices they made, recommit to the choices they made, and remember what they are most passionate about.

REFERENCES

Watson, J. (2008). *Nursing: The philosophy of science and caring.* University Press of Colorado.

13

Teaching-Learning Professional Caring Based on Jean Watson's Theory of Human Caring

Kathleen L. Sitzman, MS, RN

CARING IN NURSING

T HE BROAD CONCEPT OF "caring" has long been associated with the nursing profession. As early as the 1850s, Florence Nightingale described trained nurse caring behaviors as deliberate, holistic actions aimed at creating and maintaining an environment meant to support the natural process of healing (Nightingale, 1859). Nurse theorists and scholars have sought to describe the phenomenon of caring as it relates to professional nursing with intensified exploration of this topic starting in the late 1970s and continuing today.

Dialogue and debate about caring as it relates to nursing has resulted in differing positions among nurse scholars regarding the usefulness of identifying care as the core of nursing practice. To some, it seems that the words *care* and *caring* are so common in nursing and other disciplines, yet so vaguely understood or appreciated on a deep level, that they have lost value and meaning, becoming a bland backdrop on which to practice (Lewis, 2003). Tarlier (2004) asserted that using the terms *care* and *caring* to describe the essence, or core, of nursing are inadequate in light of the broad range of activities that nurses must engage in when

Reprinted with permission from Sitzman, K. L. (2007). Teaching-learning professional caring based on Jean Watson's Theory of Human Caring. *International Journal for Human Caring, 11*(4), 8–16.

enacting professional roles and suggested that the phrase "responsive relationships," based on ethical/moral knowledge, would be more appropriate. Watson (1985) asserted that caring is the stable *core* of all nursing activities with specific time-space limited tasks and activities comprising the continually changing *trim* of the profession.

Despite the existence of differing views, a loose consensus regarding *care* as the core of nursing arguably exists owing to the preponderance of nursing research and literature based on the notion. A general literature search, in 2007 of the EBSCO Host Research Data Bases (1975–2007), using the search words "nursing and caring," found 4,406 results. References to caring in nursing literature are so ubiquitous that it is difficult to form one inclusive definition of the term as it relates to nursing. In on-going efforts to elucidate caring as it relates to nursing, nurse theorists have created definitions that often compliment one another, serving to extend and deepen understanding of what caring is and to clarify what behaviors, attitudes, and philosophies best exemplify fully engaged professional caring across the many specialty areas found in nursing (Sitzman & Eichelberger, 2004).

Descriptions of professional caring in nursing are often based on holism and describe multiple layers of caring based on internal (philosophical) and external (scientific observable) perceptions/ feelings/actions of those who interact in caring exchanges (Boykin, Schoenhofer, Smith, St. Jean, & Aleman, 2003; Edwards, 2001; Kyle, 1995; McCance, McKenna, & Boore, 1999; Meyer & Lavin, 2005; Nelms, 1996; Patistea, 1999; Summer, 2001). The wide range of interpretations of caring in nursing literature has shown that caring means different things to different nurses, depending on amount of professional experience, level of education of the nurses involved, where and how the concept is applied, personal values, and professional focus. Throughout the completion of BSN studies, nursing students are exposed to many forms and philosophies of caring through curriculum content and interaction/socialization with practicing nurses. The concept of caring is central to the nursing discipline yet an understanding of the depth of the concept of caring often eludes nursing students and practicing nurses, owing to the widespread use of the term. The aim of a course created for senior BSN students at Weber State University (WSU) is to focus on Jean Watson's definition of caring and then assist students to enact professional caring based on a deepened understanding of this sometimes misunderstood and trivialized term.

CARING CURRICULUM WITHIN THE WEBER STATE UNIVERSITY NURSING PROGRAM

Since 1953, the curriculum in the WSU Nursing Program has consistently focused on practical, holistic caring. For the last 20 years the same four nurse theorists have formed the underpinnings of the program: Florence Nightingale, Virginia Henderson, Madeleine Leininger, and Jean Watson. All of these theorists are unique in their contributions to curriculum yet all share the focus of enacting holistic, intentional caring practices, which are core values taught throughout the WSU Nursing Program.

A course called "Integration of Professional Concepts" (N4900), required in the last semester of BSN study at WSU, is meant to help students focus on applied caring by translating theoretical caring into professional practice. Because the concept of caring is central to the WSU Nursing Program's theoretical underpinnings, the coursework in this class requires reflective evaluation of caring themes encountered throughout BSN study and serves to clarify the importance of intentional caring in professional nursing practice. Because Watson's theory of human caring philosophically encompasses archetypes of Nightingale, Henderson, and Leininger, it is the focus of this course. Deepened study, exploration, and real-world application of Watson's theory throughout the N4900 course helps students work toward building unique caring professional identities based on enhanced understanding of caring.

OVERVIEW OF JEAN WATSON'S THEORY OF HUMAN SCIENCE AND HUMAN CARE

In the mid to late 1970s, Jean Watson sought to find a common meaning for the discipline of nursing that applied to all work settings. Watson proposed that engaged professional nurses, regardless of specialty area, have awareness of the interconnectedness of all beings and share the common, intentional goal of attending to and supporting healing from both scientific and philosophical perspectives. This common goal is referred to as the caring-healing consciousness. While acknowledging the cure orientation of medicine, and nursing's legitimate place in participating in that process, Watson's theory provides balance by also identifying and describing nursing's unique carative, rather than curative, orientation in healthcare (Watson, 2007).

Watson's early theory development was organized around 10 carative factors that later evolved into the 10 clinical caring caritas processes that form the basis of the theory at the present time. The transpersonal caring moment is also central to Watson's theory. These concepts are described in greater detail below.

Ten Clinical Caritas Processes

Watson developed 10 caritas to describe fully engaged nursing practice. These processes are based on intention and mindfulness in the moment and can be effectively applied in any specialty area; during any nursing activity, for example during scientific/technical actions undertaken in critical care settings; and also during philosophical verbal exchanges between nurse and hospice client. Genuine caring exchanges are possible when the nurse mindfully enacts the following (summarized from Watson, 2007):

1. Practicing loving-kindness within the context of an intentional caring consciousness.
2. Being fully present in the moment and acknowledging the deep belief system and subjective life world of self and other.
3. Cultivating one's own spiritual practices with comprehension of inter-connectedness that goes beyond the individual.
4. Developing and sustaining helping-trusting, authentic caring relationships.
5. Being present to and supportive of the expression of positive and negative feelings arising in self and others with the understanding that all of these feelings represent wholeness.
6. Creatively using all ways of being, knowing, and caring as integral parts of the nursing process.
7. Engaging in genuine teaching-learning experiences that arise from an understanding of interconnectedness.
8. Creating and sustaining a healing environment at physical/readily observable levels and also at non-physical, subtle energy, and

consciousness levels, whereby wholeness, beauty, comfort, dignity, and peace are enabled.

9. Administering human care essentials with an intentional caring consciousness meant to enable mind-body-spirit wholeness in all aspects of care; tending to spiritual evolution of both other and self.

10. Opening and attending to spiritual-mysterious and existential dimensions of existence pertaining to self and others.

These 10 caring caritas are based on the notion that all of life is interconnected. Each self/other exchange is made up of shared energy between all who are present during the interaction. The caring nurse recognizes the evolving physical/spiritual being in the other and also recognizes and nurtures the physical/spiritual being in the self, for it is not possible to provide authentic caring to another without first being able to care for self (Sitzman & Eichelberger, 2004).

Transpersonal Caring Relationship

Transpersonal caring relationships consist of connections that embrace the spirit or soul of the other through the processes of full, authentic, caring/healing attention in the moment (Watson, 1988). Transpersonal caring implies that the nurse consciously focuses on self and other within interpersonal exchanges that are grounded in the present moment, while at the same time going beyond the moment and opening to new possibilities. The nurse values the existence of the other's inner and outer perspectives and seeks to acknowledge the connection that already exists between self and other. The authentic transpersonal caring exchange supports and augments technical care, comfort measures, pain control, sense of well-being, and transcendence of suffering. Each person in the exchange is viewed as whole and complete (Watson, 2007).

In summary, Watson's theory is about mindful, deliberate caring for self and other. Enacting Watson's theory will support fully engaged nursing practice that reflects deliberative and professionally mature/appropriate nursing actions. Caring in this sense is not a matter of *doing* caring actions in a prescriptive way to obtain desired results; rather it is an approach that advocates caring as a state of *being*.

APPLIED CARING

Because of an emphasis on philosophical concepts, Watson's theory may appear impractical and difficult to apply in everyday nursing situations but this is not necessarily so. The content in N4900 was created with the intention of clarifying what Watson's theoretical "caring" actually looks like in relation to the work of caring nurses in a variety of settings and then inspiring new BSNs to build their own action-oriented caring identities to carry out into the real world.

CONCEPTUAL ORGANIZATION OF THE COURSE

Although caring for individual clients is the most commonly accepted image in relation to caring in nursing, there are many other layers and types of caring related to nursing practice. The basic venues of caring that are explored in N4900 include caring for self, others, peers/co-workers, nursing leadership, local/world communities, the environment, and Web-based interactions. Exploring nurse activities within these venues, and identifying which of Watson's 10 caritas apply to various activities, help students make tangible connections between Watson's theoretical definitions of caring and caring expressed in daily professional practice.

BSN coursework at WSU illustrates caring activities related to self, others, peers/co-workers, leaders, local/world communities, environmental concerns, and Web-based interactions but the connection between theoretical caring and practical professional caring is often not formally discussed in class and students miss opportunities to forge deepened understandings of engaged, transpersonal caring associated with everyday nursing practice. For this reason, in the first few weeks of class, Watson's theory is explored in depth and the core content of previously completed BSN courses is revisited with the express goal of purposefully connecting Watson's theoretical concepts to content already learned. Following this, students explore the scholarly works of nurses from different disciplines that describe/demonstrate engaged caring in relation to seven different venues: self, others, peers/co-workers, nurse leaders, local/world communities, the environment, and web-based interactions. Coaching and facilitation by the instructor allow students to begin successfully identifying caritas that are applicable to each venue and to envision how they might mindfully enact transpersonal caring that is purposefully expressive of Watson's theory. To illustrate different forms of caring within each venue, examples from nursing literature are provided for the students to read and explore with classmates. In addition, students are asked to discuss which of Watson's 10 caritas might be applicable to what is described in each article. After completing all of the venue-related units of study, students create and enact a professional caring project associated with one of the venues studied in class. In the final 2 weeks of the course, students present the process and the results of their caring professional projects to each other.

CARING FOR SELF

The "Caring for the Self" unit of study discusses the importance of productively attending to multiple aspects of work and personal life. Heeding to personal and family matters, obtaining adequate rest and nutrition, engaging in stress reduction strategies, balancing home and work activities, and protecting self in the work environment all pertain to adequate self-care. An imbalance in one area typically affects all other areas of functioning. Upheaval resulting from lack of self-care can be envisioned as dropping a pebble into a still pond; ripples originate with the turmoil caused by the dropped pebble (lack of self-care) and then radiate outward until the entire pond is disturbed to varying degrees (the effect that lack of self-care has on a person's surroundings). This allegory may also be considered in a constructive light with the dropped pebble signifying deliberate self-care activities and the ripples positively energizing all that surrounds the self. Loving, caring for, and respecting self is the first step in enabling enlightened caring for others, which has the power to transform surroundings in ever-widening circles of influence. Watson (2005, p. 142) quoted an ancient Chinese proverb that illustrates this point well:

> *If there is light in the soul,*
> *There is beauty in the person.*
> *If there is beauty in the person,*
> *There is harmony in the house.*
> *If there is harmony in the house,*
> *There is order in the nation.*
> *If there is order in the nation,*
> *There will be peace in the world.*
>
> (Anonymous)

ARTICLES THAT ILLUSTRATE SELF-CARE

Foley (2004) addressed workplace safety for nurses in varied clinical settings, expressing the conviction that nurses focus on providing quality care to others and sometimes do not engage in quality self-care to avoid workplace hazards and injury: " . . . nurses must also focus on taking care of themselves so they are able to continue to provide quality care for their patients and maintain the profession's ability to recruit and retain new nurses" (Foley, p. 91). Attending to basic self-care through the preservation of safety and health among the myriad of risks present in the nursing profession supports long-term health and professional longevity.

In addition to basic preservation of safety and health, Turkel and Ray (2004) clarified the importance of caring for self holistically, saying, "The soul of nursing is seeking the good of self and others through compassionate caring. Healing and caring for oneself is vital to have the energy to compassionately care for others" (p. 249). Turkel and Ray discussed the importance of creating an organizational work culture meant to support self-care. Suggestions for enhancing self-care in the workplace included providing multiple opportunities for for-mal and informal communication; acknowledging when one nurse's engaged professional caring made a difference in the life of a colleague or client; celebrating the human spirit through posters and photographs hung in work areas; creating a calm, clean, and pleasant break room; not expecting overtime or frequent shift rotation; offering opportu-nities for participation in alternative healing therapies; and having nurses develop a plan of self-care as part of the annual evaluation and respecting implementation of the plan (Turkel & Ray).

These authors made an eloquent argument for the importance of self-care in nursing:

> Self-care highlights the greatest asset of all—the individual. Self-care is critical to health and healing. The idea of the nurse as holistic-body, mind, and spirit, was illuminated by Watson in her theory of caring. A nurse who is holistic and self-caring can create harmony with others through authentic presence in the caring moment. If one does not appreciate the self as a caring person or if the nurse does not care for self, it is impossible for her [him] to compassionately care for others. (Turkel & Ray, p. 250)

CARING FOR OTHERS

For the purposes of conceptual simplification, the "Caring for Others" unit of study is limited to the exploration of interactions with clients. Watson (1985) described caring behaviors associated with client teaching/learning, biophysical needs, intrapersonal and interpersonal needs, developmental conflicts, loss, and stress. Effectiveness of caring for others relies on mindful engagement and cultivation of connection, in the moment, initiated by the nurse. Nurses have been taught to maintain professional distance when interacting with clients, so how is it appropriate to offer the whole self when entering into caring exchanges with clients? Watson (1988) clarified this distinction:

> Nurses and other health professionals have been warned to avoid personal interactions . . . The concept of involvement as the participation of the entire self, using every dimension of the person as a resource in the professional relation, is entailed in the concept of transpersonal caring relationship between nurse and person. . . . [These relationships differ from personal relationships with friends and family because] . . . the focus of a patient's personal involvement . . . is directed toward the problem at hand and its effect upon his or her life. (pp. 64–65)

ARTICLES THAT ILLUSTRATE CARING FOR OTHERS

Askinazi (2004), an author in the process of completing an Associate's Degree in Nursing, wrote a commentary addressing caring about caring. Caring means:

> We escape our own boundaries and egos as we completely and openly focus on our patients. At the same time, our patients' personal boundaries are fraying, often because they have such a great need for physical or emotional relief. Surprisingly, this permeability ends up making each patient and nurse able to form a new connection in that space that usually separates two people. A new experience exists that is neither of the nurse nor the patient, but of both, experienced together. (Askinazi, p. 33)

This article provided perspectives from a nursing student not unlike many students in the class.

Fredriksson (1999) explored modes of relating in a caring conversation between nurse and client. Specifically, the existence or absence of in-the-moment presence, touch, and listening was addressed. The importance of intentionality in terms of being with the client in the present moment was highlighted. Touch was described as a form of relating during task-oriented, as well as interpersonal, interactions. The difference between hearing and listening was clarified with hearing being described as merely an auditory sensory phenomenon and listening being intentional connection through auditory phenomenon (Fredriksson).

INTERACTING WITH PEERS/CO-WORKERS

The "Interacting with Peers/Co-Workers" unit of study explores immediacy, mindfulness, and appreciation for interconnectedness during co-worker interactions. Peer/Co-Worker caring supports an environment that acknowledges and upholds the worth and dignity of all, including clients, significant others, peers, and interdisciplinary partners. It is difficult to engage in holistic care with clients unless co-worker interactions are consciously and deliberately enacted with attention to basic human caring needs and respect for/acknowledgement of the importance of interconnection and collaboration.

ARTICLES THAT ILLUSTRATE CARING INTERACTIONS WITH PEERS/CO-WORKERS

Daiski (2004) examined views of nurses who work in hospital settings about their professional relationships/interactions with nursing colleagues and others on the healthcare team. Daiski discussed the long-held belief that nurses engage in oppressed group behavior, which contributes to uncaring, non-supportive interactions between nurse peers. Daiski's study validated this belief:

> Nurses largely remain an oppressed group, dominated by those considered more powerful, such as physicians, who continue to intrude on nursing matters . . . the continuing subordination to those thought of as more powerful was attributed to lack of self-confidence and to a desire to please [those with power]. (p. 48)

Negative peer interactions stemmed from feelings of disempowerment due to lack of attention to and/or consideration of staff nurses' basic desire to be recognized for good work and be included in decision-making that affects them. Respondents' ideas for improvement included recognition for excellence in job performance, nurse (rather than non-nurse) mediated transition and change when needed within the organization, greater advocacy by nurse managers, and continuing education/professional development.

Hayhurst, Saylor, and Stuenkel (2005) studied perceptions of work environmental factors that supported retention of nurses. Results showed:

> Nurses who stayed reported less work pressure and greater peer cohesion, supervisor support, and autonomy than nurses who left . . . Job satisfaction among nurses has been correlated with perceived social support from their colleagues and physicians. This sense of social and collegial support may be one of the reasons nurses decided to stay at their current jobs, even though other factors might not have been ideal. (Hayhurst et al., pp. 286–287)

NURSING LEADERSHIP

The "Nursing Leadership" unit of study explores many facets of nursing leadership. Performing research is a form of nursing leadership. The creation of scholarly articles represents caring through leadership, since adding to nursing knowledge in this way shows deep caring for the nursing profession. Integrating concepts of intentional, deliberative, fully engaged professional caring into the workplace also requires nursing leadership. Caring nursing leadership may also be demonstrated through membership in professional organizations and through political action.

ARTICLES THAT ILLUSTRATE CARING IN RELATION TO NURSING LEADERSHIP

Bent and colleagues (2005) helped create caring change in a large healthcare system through action research that linked practice, theory, and inquiry in the delivery of care-centered services. The authors acknowledged that small caring moments form the underpinnings for caring as expressed throughout an organization, "Often, healing moments in our busy practices go unnoticed or are not recognized for their significance and influence on the healing environment. Honoring these moments fuels the heart with the energy to care" (Bent et al., p. 24). Goals that were formed to fuel the advancement of a caring theoretical foundation for the organization included honoring the caring practice of nurses, honoring the unique experiences and contributions of United States veterans, building a framework for strengthening nursing practice, defining caring practice and the ethical foundations of nursing, developing nursing knowledge (perform research) within a caring framework, actively articulating to others the value of nursing, and uniting nursing through a culture of caring for self and other (Bent et al.).

Ryan (2005) described integrating Jean Watson's theory of human caring into nursing practice across a multihospital care system. Watson's theory was integrated into multiple nursing functions and organizations within the system, for example:

> The nursing theory has been woven into the job description and the clinical ladder process. The nursing job descriptions now include a statement that the nurses must be competent in both technological skills and carative factors of the caring theory. Within the clinical ladder process, candidates applying for clinical advancement are interviewed . . . the candidate shares a story from their professional practice that demonstrates how they positively influenced a patient outcome. The candidate must then identify and discuss the carative factors exemplified in their story. (Ryan, p. 28)

Wesorick (2004) told a personal leadership story about caring, involving one woman's efforts to create a more caring environment in the hospital where she worked. Inspired by colleagues and the work of caring leadership, the nurse in this story begins with despair and ends with hope and resolve at the prospect of effecting positive change in support of creating a more caring workplace.

LOCAL AND WORLD COMMUNITIES

The "Caring for Local and World Communities" unit of study clarifies the point that fully engaged professional nursing care in relation to local and world communities requires understanding and skills associated with self-care, other care, effective peer interactions, and caring/

engaged leadership. The movement in nursing toward acknowledging widespread health concerns is not new. Florence Nightingale, Clara Barton, Lillian Wald, and countless other nurse leaders throughout the 19th and 20th centuries have called upon nurses to aid in community care and reform and to assume leadership roles in the care of communities—whatever the size.

ARTICLES THAT ILLUSTRATE CARING FOR LOCAL AND WORLD COMMUNITIES

Falk-Rafael (2005a) discussed the emergence of the critical caring perspective in community health nursing. Through the application of critical caring, described as a way of being, choosing, and knowing, Falk-Rafael transformed Watson's carative factors into seven carative health-promoting processes meant to form the core of public health nursing practice. The transformed carative health-promoting processes included *preparation of self* through mindful attention to societal conditions and needs; *developing and maintaining helping-trusting relationships* through appropriately addressing community needs; *incorporating a systematic, reflexive approach to caring* that embraces multiple ways of knowing along with structured, systematic approaches; *contributing to the creation of supportable, sustainable physical, social, political, and economic environments,* meaning that caring interventions and positive change are only effective if the community is able to sustain the changes after the nurse moves on to other projects; *meeting the needs and building capacity of communities and their members,* i.e., ensuring adequate infrastructure and equipping community members to eventually meet their own needs without outside assistance; and *being open and attending to spiritual-mysterious and existential dimensions* because constructing meaning from shared adversity is part of the caring process (Falk-Rafael).

Another article by Falk-Rafael (2005b) asserted that it is nursing's legacy and moral imperative to care for local and world communities. Falk-Rafael concisely stated:

> Nurses practice at the intersection of public policy and personal lives; they are, therefore, ideally situated and morally obligated to include sociopolitical advocacy in their practice. As an increasing body of literature links societal structures and relations to health, the need for nursing to fulfill its social mandate

becomes even more critical for the health of the public and the future of nursing. (p. 222)

THE ENVIRONMENT

The "Caring for the Environment" unit of study explores the notion that local and world environmental concerns deeply affect the health of self and others. Nurses work closely with people who have been affected by environmental concerns; for example, infants and children exposed to lead paint that now have neurological deficits, workers who cleared the environmentally hazardous rubble from the 2001 World Trade Center collapse who are now suffering multiple health problems, soldiers who have been exposed to chemical agents, or a worker who is deaf due to working in a factory with excessive noise levels. Nurses work closely with people who have suffered health effects from various environmental exposures and have experience with environmental health issues that others do not possess. Because of this experience, nurses should be included at the highest level of policy making. Sattler (2003a) stated:

> There should be an oncology nurse at the table when carcinogen standards are being developed, a pediatric nurse when children's environmental health regulations are being developed, and a nurse midwife when reproductive toxins are being discussed. The time is ripe, and the environmental health risksare many; nurses indeed must take their seats at the policy table. (p. 5)

ARTICLES THAT ILLUSTRATE CARING FOR THE ENVIRONMENT

Sattler (2003b) addressed environmental healthcare risks created by the healthcare industry and asserted that many of those risks are preventable. In particular, two toxins created by the hospital industry are discussed: " . . . mercury pollution, and dioxins, an unintentional by-product created by the manufacture and incineration of polyvinyl chloride plastics" (p. 6). Activities of nurses who have taken leadership roles in addressing and abating these risks were highlighted in this article.

Anderko (2003) discussed protecting the health of children through environmental health tracking. She stated, "Nursing leadership, particularly as it relates to political advocacy for continued and improved funding, is essential if one is to unlock the mysteries behind causes in the upsurge in childhood diseases" (p. 14) such as asthma and childhood cancers.

Gilden (2003) discussed community involvement at hazardous waste sites and reviewed policies from a nursing perspective. Nurses were urged to become knowledgeable about hazardous waste removal policy so they are able to advocate for patients and provide leadership to affected communities. "By understanding the policies governing cleanup of hazardous waste sites, nurses can have a vital role in ensuring communities are protected and involved in decision making" (Gilden, p. 29).

CARING IN WEB-BASED ENVIRONMENTS

The "Caring in Web-Based Environments" unit of study is included in this course because nurses must often work within web-based and/or on-line environments. Information regarding on-line etiquette is widely available and is helpful in clarifying what is thought of as considerate behavior, however understanding the phenomenon of *caring* in on-line environments is in need of further investigation. Watson (2005) addressed use of technology that increasingly defines our personal and professional interactions, saying:

> This non-linear, free-association format of hypertext, multimedia, multi-sensory juxtaposition of pictures and words creates a new form of expression: three-dimensional, colored, animated symbols for interaction versus an ordered linear text that is passively read . . . the mind-to-mind, consciousness-to-consciousness connection in the world of cyberspace creates a disembodied human-to-human connection. (p. 201)

ARTICLES THAT ILLUSTRATE CARING IN WEB-BASED ENVIRONMENTS

Simpson (2004) discussed how information technology improves nursing care through the availability of education, online performance management that allow nurses to assess efficacy of care, and mapping outcomes to practice that allows nurses to rapidly and effectively debate, create, and disseminate information related to definitions of caring in nursing. Technology allows nurses to efficiently collect data and then effectively translate that data into useful information. Simpson asserted that information technology " . . . reinforces—rather than destroys—the unique and intangible quality of caring in nursing" (p. 302).

Leners and Sitzman (2006) and Sitzman and Leners (2006) explored how on-line caring is perceived by baccalaureate and graduate nursing students. Themes associated with effective on-line caring that may be helpful in everyday nursing practice include:

- Timeliness—The nurse promptly and consistently responds to e-mails, not letting more than 48 hours pass between received messages and responses.
- Personal Connection and Empathy—Sensitivity to personal issues, periodically asking how a person is doing, and responding in a caring way when personal challenges are expressed by the sender. Sharing something of oneself, outside of the necessary job-related exchange, with established on-line colleagues may also be helpful.
- Clarity—Clear and thorough instructions for how to complete projects and requests are always provided.
- Multiple Contact Opportunities—It is important to make oneself available not only via e-mail but also via telephone and in-person appointments.

Caring Projects

After completing the units of study discussed above, students create and enact a professional caring project. During the final 2 weeks of class, students present the process and results of their caring professional projects to each other. During the presentation, they must discuss how the project was enacted, what venue the project was enacted in, and explain how the project corresponds with one or two of Watson's 10 caritas. They must also elucidate why and how the project demonstrated and/or deepened personal and professional knowledge in relation to deliberate caring. The final class day, after all members of the class have had the opportunity to present their caring projects and have benefited from hearing about the learning and discoveries of others, students are asked to reflect on what they have learned in the course and then share their thoughts in informal discussion groups. In this way, students have the opportunity to assess personal growth that has taken place over the semester and celebrate the growth and accomplishments of classmates. Examples of caring projects, corresponding venues, and applicable caritas (Watson, 2007) are listed below:

- Self-Care

  A student who was feeling burned out and exhausted with the demands of work and school decided to re-evaluate his emotional/physical/spiritual health and embark on an individualized, structured rest, exercise, and diet regime aimed at restoring emotional/spiritual engagement in work activities and increasing personal vitality.

  Watson Caritas: Cultivation of one's own spiritual practices and transpersonal self, going beyond ego self.

- Caring for Others

  One student became a senior companion for the local council on aging.

  Watson Caritas: Being authentically present, and enabling and sustaining the deep belief system and subjective life world of self and other.

- Caring Interactions with Peers/Co-Workers

  One student worked within a close-knit group in an intensive care unit that would be closed forever in 3 months due to closure of the entire hospital. The staff was grieving this loss so the student decided to take workplace photographs, record anecdotes from each of her co-workers, and then create and give out "memories" DVDs in an effort to support each peer/co-worker as they coped with the loss and grief associated with this life event.

  Watson Caritas: Opening and attending to spiritual-mysterious and existential dimensions of one's own life-death: soul care for self and the one being cared for.

- Caring Associated with Nurse Leadership
  One student interviewed a nurse manager and asked what employees could do to better support her in her role as manager, then (with the unit manager's permission) communicated the results to peers at a general staff meeting.

Watson Caritas: Developing and sustaining a helping-trusting, authentic caring relationship.

- Caring for Local/World Communities

Two students teamed up to design and create a cheerful, colorful, pediatric examination room in the local homeless shelter clinic.

Watson Caritas: Creating healing environment at all levels, physical as well as non-physical, subtle environment of energy and consciousness, whereby wholeness, beauty, comfort, dignity, and peace are potentiated.

- Caring for the Environment

Two students researched waste disposal policies in the home healthcare agency where they worked and found that there was not a policy on environmentally friendly disposal procedures for worn-out durable medical equipment (DME). These students found out where to take worn-out DME for recycling and then wrote a policy for the agency that outlined the procedure for all clinicians.

Watson Caritas: Systematic use of self and all ways of knowing as part of the caring process; to engage in artistry of caring-healing practices.

- Caring in Web-Based Environments

One student invited her classmates to participate in an on-line get-to-know-you exercise to help class mates become comfortable with the on-line portion of the class and to encourage camaraderie and fun in the on-line posting forums. Every student in the class participated in this exercise even though it was entirely optional.

Watson Caritas: Engaging in genuine teaching-learning experience that attends to unity of being and meaning attempting to stay within others' frame of reference.

OBSERVATIONS FROM THE CLASSROOM

Students often commented that they were unaware of the many layers associated with professional caring until completing the coursework for N4900. Many also voiced a commitment to continued exploration and cultivation of deliberate, informed, professional caring practices after graduation. Students often verbalized the realization that transpersonal, deep caring is not necessarily expressed in obvious, outward displays but is subtly, holistically conveyed as a result of an inward philosophical stance assumed by the one providing care. Over-whelmingly positive end-of-semester course evaluations have indicated that the content areas and class activities provided clarification and meaning related to fully understanding the act of professional caring in nursing.

CONCLUSION

Engaged professional caring involves much more than one-to-one interactions with clients. Fully engaged professional caring encompasses conscious cultivation of transpersonal interactions/connections with self, peers, and clients. It includes attention to leadership, local/world communities, environmental concerns, and Web-based interactions. Nurses work in multiple venues and interact with a wide range of individuals and groups. Cultivation of awareness regarding how to embody and convey professional caring in all aspects/venues of the profession is critical to personal/professional development and also to the continued evolution of the nursing profession toward a common identity with caring at the core. The N4900 course described offers one way to help senior BSN students enter the nursing profession with a deeper understanding of, and a stronger appreciation for, the power of engaged, deliberate, theoretically based caring professional practice.

REFERENCES

Anderko, L. (2003). Protecting the health of our nation's children through environmental health tracking. *Policy, Politics, & Nursing Practice, 4*(1), 14–21.

Askinazi, A. (2004). Caring about caring. *Nursing Forum, 39*(2), 33–34.

Bent, K. N., Burke, J. A., Eckman, A., Hottmann, T., McCabe, J., & Williams, R. N. (2005). Being and creating caring change in a healthcare system. *International Journal for Human Caring, 9*(3), 20–25.

Boykin, A., Schoenhofer, S. O., Smith, N., St. Jean J., & Aleman, D. (2003). Transforming practice using a caring-based nursing model. *Nursing Administration Quarterly, 27*(3), 223–230.

Daiski, I. (2004). Changing nurses' disempowering relationship patterns. *Journal of Advanced Nursing, 48*(1), 43–50.

Edwards, S. D. (2001). Benner and Wrubel on caring in nursing. *Journal of Advanced Nursing, 33*(2), 167–171.

Falk-Rafael, A. (2005a). Advancing nursing theory through theory-guided practice: The emergence of a critical caring perspective. *Advances in Nursing Science, 28*(1), 38–49.

Falk-Rafael, A. (2005b). Speaking truth to power: Nursing's legacy and moral imperative. *Advances in Nursing Science, 28*(3), 212–223.

Foley, M. (2004). Caring for those who care: A tribute to nurses and their safety. *Online Journal of Issues in Nursing, 9*(3), 91–103.

Fredriksson, L. (1999). Modes of relating in caring conversation: A research synthesis on presence. *Journal of Advanced Nursing, 30*(5), 1167–1176.

Gilden, R. C. (2003). Community involvement at hazardous waste sites: A review of policies from a nursing perspective. *Policy, Politics, & Nursing Practice, 4*(1), 29–35.

Hayhurst, A., Saylor, C., & Stuenkel, D. (2005). Work environmental factors for the retention of nurses. *Journal of Nursing Care Quality, 20*(3), 283–288.

Kyle, T. V. (1995). The concept of caring: A review of the literature. *Journal of Advanced Nursing, 21*(4), 506–514.

Leners, D., & Sitzman, K. (2006). Graduate student perceptions: Feeling the passion of caring online. *Nursing Education Perspectives, 27*(6), 315–319.

Lewis, S. M. (2003). Caring as being in nursing: Unique or ubiquitous. *Nursing Science Quarterly, 16*(1), 37–43.

McCance, T. V., McKenna, H. P., & Boore, J. R. P. (1999). Caring: Theoretical perspectives of relevance to nursing. *Journal of Advanced Nursing, 30*(6), 1388–1395.

Meyer, G., & Lavin, M. A. (2005). Vigilance: The essence of nursing. *Online Journal of Issues in Nursing, 10*(3), 38–51.

Nelms, T. P. (1996). Living a caring presence in nursing: A Heideggerian hermeneutical analysis. *Journal of Advanced Nursing, 24*(3), 368–374.

Nightingale, F. (1859). *Notes on nursing: What it is and what it is not.* Philadelphia: Lippincott, Williams, and Wilkins.

Patistea, E. (1999). Nurses' perceptions of caring as documented in theory and research. *Journal of Clinical Nursing, 8*(5), 487–495.

Ryan, L. A. (2005). The journey to integrate Watson's caring theory with clinical practice. *International Journal for Human Caring, 9*(3), 26–30.

Sattler, B. S. (2003a). Environmental health. *Policy, Politics, and Nursing Practice, 4*(1), 4–5.

Sattler, B. S. (2003b). The greening of health care: Environmental policy and advocacy in the healthcare industry. *Policy, Politics, and Nursing Practice, 4*(1), 6–13.

Simpson, R. L. (2004). The softer side of technology: How IT helps nursing care. *Nursing Administration Quarterly, 28*(4), 302–305.

Sitzman, K., & Eichelberger, L. (2004). *Understanding the work of nurse theorists: A creative beginning.* Sudbury, MA: Jones and Bartlett Publishers.

Sitzman, K., & Leners, D. (2006). Student perceptions of caring in online baccalaureate education. *Nursing Education Perspectives, 27*(5), 254–259.

Sumner, J. (2001). Caring in nursing: A different interpretation. *Journal of Advanced Nursing, 35*(6), 926–932.

Tarlier, D. S. (2004). Beyond caring: The moral and ethical bases of responsive nurse-patient relationships. *Nursing Philosophy, 5*(3), 230–241.

Turkel, M. C., & Ray, M. A. (2004). Creating a caring practice through self-renewal. *Nursing Administration Quarterly, 28*(4), 249–254.

Watson, J. (1985). *Nursing: Human science and human care.* New York: National League for Nursing.

Watson, J. (1988). *Nursing: Human science and human care: A theory of nursing.* New York: National League for Nursing.

Watson, J. (2005). *Caring science as sacred science.* Philadelphia: F. A. Davis Company.

Watson, J. (2007). *Watson's caring theory website.* Retrieved February 5, 2007, from http://www2.uchsc.edu/son/caring/content/default.asp

Wesorick, B. (2004). A leadership story about caring. *Nursing Administration Quarterly, 28*(4), 271–275.

IV
BEYOND EVALUATION
TO AUTHENTICATION

I N THIS UNIT, WE EXPLORE different aspects of evaluating students'
performance. From a Caring Science perspective this becomes
an onerous task because the evaluation strategies used must be
congruent with the Caring Science paradigm. Although it is recognized
that teachers have the responsibility to assess students' abilities,
competencies, and knowledge, among other attributes, there has not
been significant development in this area.

The unit contains one chapter that offers a Connoisseurship model
of evaluation. We describe this model, explore the issue of grading,
and provide some examples of alternative strategies for assessing both
classroom and clinical evaluation.

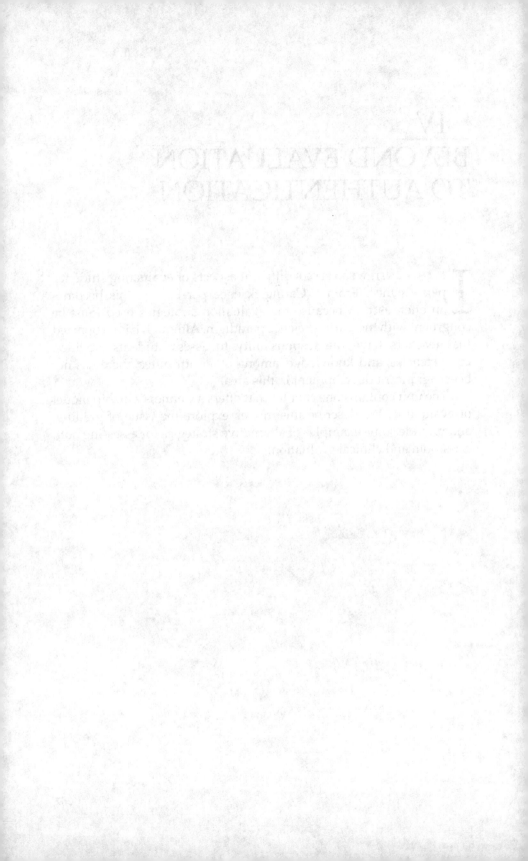

14

Connoisseurship: An Alternative Approach to Evaluation

It is through and by these means of education many of us believe
that individuals can be provoked to reach beyond themselves
into their intersubjective space. It is through and by means
of education that they can become empowered to think about
what they are doing, to become mindful, to share meanings,
to conceptualize, to make varied sense of their lived worlds . . .
—Greene, 1988, p. 12

E VALUATING STUDENT PERFORMANCE IS AN intrinsic aspect of being a teacher. Within a Caring Science curriculum, this task becomes extremely important because, if the evaluation strategies that are implemented are not congruent with the Caring Science paradigm, the evaluation process has the potential to undo all the work that preceded it. Because of the value base of a Caring Science curriculum, teachers must pay diligent attention to how students are evaluated. The evaluation strategies to be used cannot undermine the efforts of the faculty members to establish equitable, respectful, caring relations throughout a program of studies. The purpose of this chapter is to explore the issues of evaluation, grading, and assessing clinical performance and to describe some evaluation strategies that we believe are congruent with the Caring Science paradigm.

EVALUATION

Generally, evaluation is used to provide landmarks or points of reference for teachers and students. Evaluation provides indicators that let teachers and students know where they are in relation to where they want to be or where they are trying to go. Also, evaluation is a method that is used to determine worth or value, and it provides clues about progress, performance, achievement, or the lack of it. Unfortunately, all too often, evaluation becomes the most important aspect; it becomes the end instead of the means and, as a result, it can become the *driver* of the educational pursuit rather than *markers* for learning progress (Bevis, 2000, p. 265). When this occurs as it often does, everything else becomes less important and the entire learning process becomes consumed with the evaluation of learning rather than the learning itself. Because of our tendency to think of learning as behavioral change, our evaluation strategies tend to reflect this focus by attempting to measure changes in behavior. When we do this, we automatically and sometimes unknowingly, endorse a very narrow view of learning that basically says that all learning is behavioral and therefore measurable. But much of learning in nursing is *not* behavioral and therefore cannot be measured this way.

In a Caring Science curriculum based in an emancipatory relational pedagogy, we are interested in cultivating a disciplined scholarship that is necessary for developing expertise. For example, we are interested in students' abilities to "acquire insights, see patterns, find meanings and significance, see balance and wholeness, make compassionate and wise judgments, while acquiring foresight, generate creative flexible strategies, develop informed skilled intentionality, identify with ethical and cultural traditions of the field, grasp the deeper structures of the knowledge base enlarge the ability to think critically and creatively and find pathways to new knowledge" (Bevis, 2000, p. 265). Therefore, we need to develop new evaluation strategies that can access students' thinking and that can capture more of the essence of the essential attributes of a Caring Science curriculum.

CONNOISSEURSHIP

Bevis and Watson (1989) created an interpretative-criticism model of evaluation. In their model, "students are engaged with teachers in the process of criticism as a way to assist them to use knowledge and experience to make comparisons and be critics" (p. 24). We have developed this model of evaluation further and emphasize a Connoisseurship model of evaluation.

Eisner (1972) speaks of the art of appreciation that he labels *connoisseurship*. As he explains, "A connoisseur goes further than generalizations or classifications by perceiving the unique attributes of phenomena that distinguish one thing from another even within a category" (quoted in Bevis & Watson, 1989, p. 286). For teachers to use this approach to evaluation, they must have an expert grasp on: the meaning of the experience in the field; the deeper structures of the subject; the history and historically significant issues of the field; both classical and the current literature of the field; the characteristics of the educated expert nurse; the educative processes that shape the expert professional nurse; and the modes of inquiry appropriate to the field (Bevis, 1989). This evaluation model of connoisseurship focuses on developing skills of observation, critique, and authentication. These skills of connoisseurship encourage students to grow professionally and improve their expertise in nursing.

This connoisseurship model of evaluation requires a certain level of expertise and scholarship in order to provide the rich descriptions, interpretations, comparisons, and judgments that are inherent in the model. Indeed, it is precisely this experience and scholarship that distinguishes the one who is learning from the one who is evaluating the learning. So, a critical aspect of the connoisseurship approach to evaluation is the ability to teach the process of connoisseurship and criticism to the co-learners by providing them with experiences and working with them to hone their abilities to recognize *good practice*. It is not possible for students to become connoisseurs while they are students; however, as Bevis suggests, what they can do is begin an apprenticeship in the art of perception, appreciation, and comparison. "It is the very lack of experience on the part of students that handicaps them in developing 'taste' and sophistication in perceiving and interpreting events of care" (Bevis, 1989, p. 284). Bevis and Watson outline a five-part evaluation model of interpretive-criticism; we have adapted this model to consist of five parts by combining looking and seeing as *observing*. The five components of the connoisseurship model of evaluation are:

Observing—Observing requires that we both look and see. Looking at something is quite different from seeing something. "Seeing is looking with attention and focus. Seeing is attending to the details, the context, the situation, the environment, the parts, and the whole" (p. 288). It also involves recognizing what is being looked at.

Perceiving and Intuiting—Perceiving and intuiting involve our personal sensing and interpreting. Bevis and Watson distinguish this from meaning making in perception and suggest that "perception translates perceiving into experience" (p. 288). This type of perceiving requires intuition and imagination. It is similar to what Benner and Wrubel (1982) observed in expert nurses' practices. These nurses were able to perceive whole situations and know what to do in a given situation without breaking the situation down into component parts. Perceiving and intuiting in this way "involves an ability to perceive what is significant and what is trivial in a situation, a judgment that can only be made in the light of experience" (Bevis & Watson, 1989, p. 289). Working with learners to examine the significance of what they see educates them in developing their perceiving and intuiting abilities and enhances their expert judgment.

> *Rendering*—"Rendering is a way of describing the ineffable . . . it has virtual rather than actual meaning and depends upon symbolic language" (p. 290). These are thick, rich descriptions that are situation based, contextual, and subjective. They rely on the observer's ability to use metaphor, prose, imagery, and simile to give accounts of human experiences.
>
> *Interpreting Meaning*—Meanings are our personal interpretations of events. As discussed in an earlier section, they are deeply personal, and based on our assumptions, beliefs, values, and ethics. In evaluation situations, accessing students' meanings assists in understanding what they are doing with information, knowledge, and experiences.
>
> *Judging*—Judging is value based and requires that you have the context and knowledge for comparisons.

LEARNING ACTIVITY:
USING THE CONNOISSEURSHIP MODEL TO ACCESS LEARNING

Ends in View

In this learning activity, you will use the criticism and connoisseurship model to access learning.

Read

Bevis and Watson (1989). *Toward a caring curriculum: A new pedagogy for nursing*, pp. 283–287.

Write

Consider your recent clinical experience. Using the criticism and connoisseurship framework proposed by Bevis and Watson (1989) and described above, assess your clinical experience. Consider each component and evaluate your learning in your clinical experience.

Dialogue

Share your assessments of your learning experiences with your classmates. Consider the following questions:

How does this model of evaluation fit with your views of evaluation?

To what degree is this model congruent with human science pedagogy?

Reflect

In your journal, write about how you might do your practicum differently if you were to start over. Use the criticism and connoisseurship model to describe the aspects that you might focus on differently.

LEARNING ACTIVITY:
DEVELOPING CRITERIA FOR EVALUATING LEARNING

Ends in View

In this learning activity, you will have opportunities to develop criteria to assess learning.

Write

Read the following situations and choose one to work on, or you may choose a situation from your own experience if you wish. Develop criteria to assess learning, and describe how you would evaluate the situation that you have chosen. Consider how you will know that learning has taken place. What will you take as evidence that learning has occurred?

(Continued)

Situations

1. You are a nurse teaching prenatal classes. This is your final session.

2. You are in charge of continuing education and have organized a teaching/learning session on continuous patient records.

3. You are a nurse on a maternity ward and are teaching a first-time mom to bath her baby.

4. You work on a cardiac unit, and you are doing discharge planning with a 65-year-old male who is recovering from a myocardial infarction.

5. You are a community health nurse making a home visit to an elderly gentleman with diabetes.

6. You work with the Ministry of Health and have just completed a teaching/learning session on community participation in health care with the regional health officers.

Dialogue

Share the situation you chose, the criteria you developed, and the evaluation process you described with your classmates. What important points need to be remembered when developing criteria for assessing learning? What patterns emerged from the discussion of your evaluation processes? Discuss any discrepancies and examine these in relation to the Foundation of Caring Science outlined in Chapter 1.

Reflect

In your journal, reconsider the criteria you developed and the evaluation process that you described in light of your discussions with your learning partners or study group. Are there any changes you would make?

ASSESSING STUDENTS' PERFORMANCE: THE DILEMMA OF GRADING

Grading is perhaps the most difficult aspect of teaching/learning within a Caring Science paradigm. The notion of a person assigning grades to another person's work without that person being involved in the decision-making process violates the basic assumptions upon which the paradigm rests. Yet, you may find yourself in situations in which you are required to *grade* someone else's work. Usually, institutions require teachers to assign grades to students work and to submit them.

Learning and grading can be confused. It is often assumed that a grade that a student received in a course is a reflection of the learning that the student experienced in that course. Yet, we have all had experiences where we have learned a great deal but were unable to demonstrate that learning in the specific tasks (assignments) that we were asked to complete! We believe that it is important to separate learning from grading. In our opinion, learning is a deeply personal experience that has to do with the discovery of personal meaning. Grading, in contrast, is an assessment that teachers are required to make about students' performance on a set of specific tasks at a given moment in time. We are committed to having assignments relate to students' learning as much as possible, that is, to making them practical and relevant. However, in the end, it still comes down to the judgment that the teacher must make about the student's ability to meet certain criteria. In a book on curriculum development within a Caring Science paradigm, it seems even more critical that the evaluation methods be congruent with and reflect the philosophy of this paradigm. Conditions must be such that the evaluation methods used do not sabotage the integrity of the learning within a course. This means the evaluation process must be transparent and certain conditions must exist, including:

- power differences between teachers and learners are discussed and negotiated;
- criteria for evaluation are consistent with human science pedagogy;
- as much as possible, students and teachers negotiate the evaluation process;
- evaluation criteria integrate lived experiences, theoretical understandings, and critical reflection;
- peer and self-evaluation are valued.

Time Out for Reflection

Think about different ways that you have been evaluated in an education system. Answer the following questions:

What methods of evaluation stand out for you as being participatory?

Have you had an experience in which you felt that the power differential between you and the teacher was negotiated. Describe this experience.

What was your most rewarding evaluation experience?

What would you recommend as the most appropriate strategies for evaluating nursing students in a Caring Curriculum?

Contract Grading: An Alternative to Traditional Evaluation Strategies

Contract grading is an interesting strategy for evaluating students' performance that recognizes the power differences between students and teachers and then attempts to negotiate that power by allowing students to be involved in the grading process. Contract grading allows students to make important choices about what, how, and when to learn, thereby facilitating the development of a partnership learning/teaching environment. As an evaluation strategy, it is consistent with a Caring Science curriculum and an emancipatory relational pedagogy.

Contract grading can take many forms. Typically, teachers outline expectations for students for each grade level and students enter a contract for the grade that they want to achieve in the course (Table 14.1). For each grade, the number and the quality of the assignments vary. For example, if a student negotiates for a B, they do the work required for a B grade, and it must be in keeping with the quality description of a B assignment. Usually, teachers retain the discretion of assigning the plus or minus to the work produced.

To be successful, contract grading requires an up-front investment by the teacher and is initially time consuming to implement. Students are not usually familiar with this evaluation strategy and can be leery of it. Teachers need to provide as much information as possible and spend the time required to allow the students to make an informed decision about whether or not they want to participate in the contract grading evaluation. Ultimately, it is the students' collective choice that determines whether or not contract grading will be used to assess their performance. It often surprises us how students are reluctant to engage in this evaluation method. However, when you have an open discussion about the power issues involved while making it clear that

TABLE 14.1   Example Description of Teacher's Expectations for Each Grade Level

TASK	C	B	A
1. Regular attendance	Required	Required	Required
2. Journal notes	Required	Required	Required
3. Completion of two typescripts including analysis and feedback from your partner	Required	Required	Required
4. Audio or videotaped demonstration of helping interview	Required	Required	Required
5. Class presentation		Required	Required
6. Personal guidelines for helping		Required	Required
7. Research paper			Required
8. Option: (except for number 4 above). You may propose a substitution for any of the tasks listed above. This must be negotiated with the instructor. Such negotiation must be completed by July 22.			

if you evaluate them in the traditional way you have all the power, they typically engage quickly. Grade contracts do shift the power difference and help students to have more responsibility for their grades. In most cases, the teacher will have them sign an actual *contract* that does not have any weight per se but instead is a symbolic act.

One criticism of contract grading is the belief that all students should be striving for an "A." Obviously, we do not want to encourage students to strive for a D or an F as both of these are below average and failing. However, when the consequences of this choice are described to the students they usually do not choose to be unsuccessful or fail. Allowing students to retain control and responsibility for their actions is a powerful experience that enacts a Caring Science and emancipatory relational pedagogy. Putting control in the students' hands often results in their delivering better quality work. As a teacher, you need to consider the composition of your class recognizing that this might in fact give some students permission to do less. However, at the same time, other students who feel disempowered by grading might become motivated by the control they receive through grade contracts and make a better grade.

When using contract grading, a clear description of each task must be provided, and the precise criteria for grading must be described fully.

> ### LEARNING ACTIVITY:
> #### DESIGNING EVALUATION CONSISTENT
> #### WITH CARING SCIENCE CURRICULUM
>
> ### Ends in View
>
> In this learning activity, you will have an opportunity to develop your own evaluation methods that are consistent with Caring Science curriculum and an emancipatory relational pedagogy.
>
> ### Write
>
> In your journal, make a list of the characteristics that you consider to be essential to quality evaluation practices in a Caring Science curriculum. Use the list of characteristics of Caring Science pedagogy to critique these characteristics for consistency with the paradigm.
>
> ### Dialogue
>
> Share your list of characteristics of quality evaluation practices with your classmates. Compare your lists and search for common characteristics. Discuss any characteristics that do not seem to fit with your understanding.
>
> ### Reflect
>
> In your journal, illustrate how evaluation relates to other aspects of your emancipatory relational pedagogy.

CLINICAL EVALUATION:
ACCESSING STUDENTS' LEARNING

Historically nurses' clinical competence has been assessed using behavioral objectives and professional competencies. Basically, we relied on the students' ability to recite signs and symptoms of diseases, develop nursing care plans, and recall on demand the nursing care required for a particular disease. However, "behavioral objectives as guides to evaluation support a philosophy of evaluation that is reductionistic, mechanistic, control and predictive-oriented, empirical, and manipulative" (Bevis, 2000, p. 273). As we embrace Caring Science as the foundation for nursing curriculum and an emancipatory relational pedagogy, we need to develop new ways of evaluating students that are congruent with this paradigm. Clinical evaluation presents particular challenges because we need to feel comfortable that our students and graduates are safe. In the past, we tended to assume that behavioral objectives that were measurable ensured safe nursing practice. However, with only a moment's reflection, it is apparent that the tool that has always been used to assess students' clinical performance is the teacher. We rely on our judgment to assess students' abilities to practice safely. "Safety is more than performing the technical skill without error and harm to the patient. Safety also resides in being able to depart rule-driven behavior quickly, to cut through distracters to the heart of the problem and to solve it creatively (Bevis, 2000, p. 276). In this way, knowledge, understanding, insights, and intuition used wisely also determine safety, and it is to these attributes that we must turn to assess students' performance.

We turned our attention to these attributes in a study (Hills, 2000) that was designed to develop a way of evaluating clinical performance that was consistent with a Caring Science curriculum with an emancipatory relational pedagogy. We began by considering Benner's domains of practice and competencies and massaged those to be more congruent with our curriculum. We ensured that all domains and competencies were: nursing concepts not biomedical ones; included community settings as well as acute care settings; reflected health promotion; and, finally, concentrated on developing competencies that reflected what *could* be rather than what *is*. Thus, began the development of a Clinical Appraisal Form.

With consultation from several nurse scholars (Jean Watson, Em Bevis, and Chris Tanner), five domains of practice were identified: health and healing, teaching/learning, clinical judgment, professional development, and collaborative leadership. Within each domain, several quality indicators were identified with specific indicators developed for each domain that reflected changes in course themes. For example, in semester two the focus is on people's experience with chronic health challenges; thus, all of the quality indicators reflect this theme. The five domains of practice remained constant in every semester throughout the program. The quality indicators changed in each semester reflecting the semester focus and the increased complexity of learning nursing practice.

Initially, faculty members experienced difficulty using this appraisal form. "They reported a tendency to use the quality indicators outlined in the form as if they were behavioral objectives" (Hills, 2000, p. 3). Given that this form was developed specifically to replace behavioral objectives, more development was needed.

This experience led us to develop what we called the Iterative Review and Dialogue Process (Hills et al., 1993). Through our discussions, we realized that we needed to have learning and evaluation connected. Rather than *testing* students in clinical situations, we needed to access their thinking about clinical situations. We needed to access students' thinking and the way that they processed information. We know that telling stories, or narrative accounts from practice, is an effective way of accessing students thinking about clinical situations. Having them reflect on these narratives develops insight and reflective practice. The following processes were the result of many discussions and consultations.

Iterative Review and Dialogue process:

- Students write a narrative account of practice in their journal.
- Students analyze this "story" using a framework designed for this purpose.
- The story and analysis are submitted to faculty member for review.
- Faculty member responds to students' critiques by posing questions that encourage the student to further reflect on the experiences they described.
- These notes, questions, and comments are returned to the student.
- The student responds to the faculty's comments.

This iterative process is repeated.

An example of this iterative process is reflected in the journal of a first-year student who, in her second semester (people's experience with chronic health challenges), is working with a woman who is living with Parkinson's disease. She states:

> Another quality indicator of the health and healing domain
> is *beginning to develop an open caring approach*. I think this was
> illustrated when I took a seat near my client's bed so that we

could communicate openly and comfortably with each other. She welcomed this. She very much guided the communication, willingly telling me her stories of her family and her disease. I contributed by listening. A question posed to me was "what is it like to listen to another?". Well in this case it was very easy because I was deeply interested in her story. I tried to remain aware of my posture, keeping it as welcoming to communication as possible, which I found a little difficult to do upon the first time meeting someone. However, my client made it easier for me because of her openness, sincerity, and her willingness to teach. I very much appreciated this. This made it extra interesting and intrigued me to listen very actively—with all my senses. I truly empathized with this woman and I could feel her frustration, her sadness, her happiness, her acceptance. I was drawn in by her knowledge, and her experience—her life. I learned so much. I tried to understand as much as I could. I did not judge or jump to conclusions. She led the way, and I followed willingly down her life's path. I was very involved.

This excerpt demonstrates how the domains of practice and the quality indicators prompt students to reflect on their clinical experiences and identify specific ways they engaged in those clinical situations. It also demonstrates how the teacher prompts the student to reflect further by asking critical questions. The iterative process is also well demonstrated in this excerpt.

Another quality indicator in the heath and healing domain is that it "focuses on the person not the disease." In this case, the student states:

I see my client just like anyone else. She is conscious of her weight, her appearance—how her hair looks. She has good days and bad days. She has interests of her own—reading. She is a person, a whole person, her own unique person, and I feel lucky to have gotten to know her the way I have. It is a wonderful, connecting experience. She was asked, "What made you mention that you see your client like just like everyone else?" The student responds:

The reason that I touched on the fact, in my story, that I see my client like anyone else is because I have heard all too often, in the past, clients being seen or known as their disease and nothing else. I have heard caregivers referring to patients as "the leg" or "the arm," depending on the client's condition.

These caregivers are neglecting to see the whole person. Some may wonder why with all those problems, such as a progressive disease, one would worry about their appearance. Again, they are neglecting to tend to the whole person, and neglecting to support their client's coping mechanisms, values, interests, and worth. I just wanted to make it clear that I don't think that way, or conduct my practice that way. Even though my client has a disease, she is more than that. She cares, hopes, copes, and dreams. She has her own special interests, and each person living with a disease has their own story. You cannot treat every Parkinson patient the same, because they are more than a Parkinson patient, they are their own unique person.

Again, the domains and competencies provide a structure for students to describe their experiences and reflections. Teachers gain access to the students' thinking and can prompt further insight and reflection by asking questions and sharing their perceptions.

New ways of evaluating clinical performance must be developed if we are to successfully shift to a Caring Science paradigm. Benner (1984) revolutionary work on excellence in clinical expertise could make a remarkable contribution to the evaluation of nursing students' clinical performance. If the concepts revealed in much of her research, but particularly in her book, *From Novice to Expert* (1984), were experimented with as guides for clinical evaluation, this contribution would be realized. As she explains:

> perceptual awareness is central to good nursing judgment and ... this begins with vague hunches and global assessments that initially bypass critical analysis; conceptual clarity follows more often than it precedes. Expert nurses often describe their perceptual abilities using phrases such as "gut feeling", a "sense of uneasiness", or "feeling that things just are not right". This kind of talk makes educators and clinicians uncomfortable, because the assessment must move from the perceptual beginnings to conclusive evidence. Expert nurses know that in all cases definitive evaluation of a patient's condition requires more than vague hunches, but through experience they have learned to allow their perceptions to lead to confirming evidence." (Benner, 1984, p. xviii–xix)

Imagine if we began to create evaluation strategies that concentrated on assessing students' abilities to recognize salient contextual features of a given clinical situation and assisted them to link this perceptual awareness to nursing actions. We would be on a new path of clinical evaluation: one that would mean that nurses were learning how to be experts and connoisseurs of their own practice, and evaluation would encourage this development, rather than act as an impediment to it.

REFERENCES

Benner, P. (1984). *From novice to expert: Excellence and power in clinical nursing practice.* London: Addison Wesley.

Benner, P., & Wrubel, J. (1982). Skilled clinical knowledge: The value of perceptual awareness, part 1. *The Journal of Nursing Administration, 12*(5), 11–14.

Bevis, E. (2000). Accessing learning: Determining worth or developing excellence—from a behaviorist toward an interpretive-criticism model. In E. Bevis & J. Watson (Eds.), *Toward a caring curriculum: A new pedagogy for nursing.* Boston: Jones & Bartlett.

Bevis, E., & Watson, J. (Eds.). (1989). *Toward a caring curriculum: A new pedagogy for nursing.* New York: National League for Nursing.

Eisner, E. (1972). Emerging models for education evaluation. *School Review, 80*(4), 573–589.

Greene, M. (1988). *The dialectic of freedom.* New York: Teacher's College Press.

Hills, M. (2000). Co-operative inquiry: Transforming clinical evaluation. In P. Reason & H. Bradbury (Eds.), *Handbook for action research.* London: Sage.

Hills, M., Belliveau, D., Calnan, R., Clarke, C., Greene, E., & Tanner, C. (1993). *An iterative dialogue process for clinical evaluation.* Unpublished manuscript.

V

ENSURING THE FUTURE OF NURSING: EMBRACING CARING SCIENCE

I N THIS LAST UNIT, WE enter into new space where we reflect and re-vision education generally. We offer another level of philosophical and ethical critique grounded in another turn of whole person, unitary consciousness—bringing the parts and whole together; bringing the heart and mind together—*educare*—the soul of education with caring. We introduce the notion of *Caritas* education—of learning and teaching, as an evolved ethic, epistemology, and pedagogy, which unites Caring and Love (Palmer, 2004).

Here we ask new questions, rhetorical and otherwise, such as what kind of curriculum can sustain *Caritas*: Love and epistemology and pedagogy as ethic? How do we break the dominant mind-set of separation and put the parts back into the whole?

We seek to reconcile and unify educational, epistemological, and ethical models of caring as pedagogical and curricular reforms now and in the future—for nursing education, science, and society alike.

In this closing unit we consider transformational learning concepts and introduce broader energetic symbolic notions of "words"—words we use in teaching, learning, theories, and interpretations, in communicating our knowing, being, doing. We reveal how "words" and language carry energetic power to influence others, for better or for worse.

Language, combined with the power of personal experiences, possesses the energy of love and caring. Thus we seek to address the "ethics of face" of the individual, as unique "other," whether in the classroom or clinical setting, near or afar, real time or virtual, reaffirming that Caring Science is not a unitary singular rule-bound approach. Rather, Caring Science invites all the diversity and synergistic emergence of science, arts, philosophy, and humanities, with personal meaning, growth, and evolving consciousness—awakening to an expanding and changing worldview that is upon us.

Finally we conclude by proposing "Authentication Criteria with examples of 'Disciplinary Evidence' relevant for a Caring Science Curriculum"; for example, what would be/could be some operational and philosophical guidelines for anyone considering taking this disciplinary Caring Science curriculum perspective seriously?

These new authentication criteria can be the rhetorical over riding evidentiary directions for all futuristic programs. They incorporate distinct Caring Science *disciplinary* criteria as an evolved standard and evidence-guide to help assure and sustain nursing as a distinct caring-healing-health discipline and profession for another century.

15
Reflecting and Re-visioning: Bringing the Heart and Mind Together

To take love seriously and to bear and to learn it like a task, this
is what people need. For one human being to love another, that
is perhaps the most difficult of all our tasks, the ultimate, the
last test and proof, the work for which all other work is but a
preparation.
—*Rainer Maria Rilke*

BRINGING THE HEART AND MIND TOGETHER FOR *CARITAS* (CARING AND LOVE) EDUCATION

I t is acknowledged that it takes about 100 years for a profession to mature as a distinct separate entity and come of age in its own right. As we complete this book, we honor and acknowledge this year, 2010, as the centenary of Florence Nightingale, the founder of modern nursing in the world, who died in 1910. Thus, we are here together 100 years later, to make the right choices for this historic timeline and to reignite the enduring light and love of the heart and soul of nursing's human caring knowing/being/doing in the world.

Because nursing and nursing education are at a critical turning point for survival, due to all the conflicting demands, nursing and nurse educators are invited to make the hard turn toward its disciplinary foundation, in what we have posed as Caring Science. This work both honors the past and opens a new horizon for an inspired future of nursing for sustaining human caring around the globe throughout time.

This chapter draws heavily upon Watson, J. 2008a: Chapter 20, pp. 245–261 (excerpts used with permission of University Press of Colorado).

Without making the hard mature turn to be directly accountable to the public for its Caring Science disciplinary foundation, as a
continuous, constantly evolving guide to mature caring-healing-health
knowledge and practices, nurses may succumb to being very good
technicians of a totally transformed health-care system. If that were
to occur, nursing will have lost its way and the path embedded in
its ancient and noble history. In continuing the evolutionary turn toward Caring Science as the disciplinary foundation to guide future
practices, nursing continues to evolve in harmony with the evolution
of human consciousness and its global covenant with society and
humanity itself.

*As we bring closure to this work, we also open our hearts to time-
less and rhetorical questions which haunt us through the ages. As
nursing educators and as a caring profession, where are we to learn the
ultimate, the last test and proof of the work of humanity with which we
deal: Human Caring/*Caritas*/Love and our shared human conditions?

Native Americans and indigenous cultures around the globe
offer insights and wisdom beyond our extant mythic epistemology.
Their unitary, whole-worldview approach to knowing is by honoring
human life within the context of a comprehensive cosmology that
informs views of life and death, living and dying, and humans' place
in the universe. In their cosmology, life and death, knowledge, and
all of life's events are one great sacred circle of the web of life. Real
life, health, and illness stories of healing, survival, changing, dying are
beyond humans' full control; they have to be considered within the
web of life itself, from a wiser knowledge system, a larger cosmology, a
larger ethic than our rational, ego, cognitive, lens. This shift to a larger
cosmology that integrates Caring and Love and Healing is essential if
we are to sustain humanity for both human and planetary survival at
this point in history (Levinas, 1969).

This is a time in our human history to put the parts back into the
whole, toward a living ethic, epistemology, and ontology of wholeness, relationship, and human caring–healing. It is a time for education, for curriculum, for teaching and learning to serve the evolution of
our shared humanity and our common tasks for surviving and thriv-
ing in an unfolding and dramatically changing world and Planet.

We can say that Caring Science is a model of thought and practice in
which biomedical science and technical evidence alone are not simply

---

* This section draws upon the work of Watson (2005).

blended with *Caritas* but that biomedical science and evidence per se are subsumed within an ethical dimension as the prime consideration; a dimension that recognizes "the face of other," beyond "any case."

In this respect, we assert that "Caring Science" can be defined as "an evolving ethical-epistemic field of study that is grounded in the discipline of nursing and informed by related fields; as such, it incorporates Love as a core element of human-human-divine connections" (Watson & Smith, 2002, p. 456).

The fact that nursing deals with phenomena of human caring, relationships, health-illness, living, dying, pain, suffering, and all the vicissitudes of human existence, forces nursing education and practice to acknowledge and further develop an expanded view of science. We offer a science model that can accommodate Love and all of humanity. You may ask, How can we dare to put an illusive concept such as Love in a model of science? On the other hand, we reply: how can we dare not to include Love in its fullest sense in our science, since Love is core to sustaining humanity, human caring, and learning.

This view has obvious implications for the future of nursing education and practice and indeed invites challenges for nursing as a caring profession; it also offers a fresh futuristic vision for an educational ethos that would seek to promote this ethic of "face," of Love, of relation and connection with all. To reference Levinas, "the face" of other answers to "the unquenchable desire for infinity" (1969, p.150). At the same time, this separate other yet "presence of 'the face' [of other] includes all the possibilities of the transcendent relationship" (p. 155). This understanding helps us make new connections between Levinas's notion of "the face" and the transcendence of transpersonal caring—a welcoming of "the face" in a caring moment, connecting with the infinite field of universal Love in the moment (Watson, 2005), whether in the classroom or clinical setting.

With this understanding, Levinas's views take us, in education and practice, beyond the purely scientific model back to the face and the inexhaustible dimensions of our shared humanity in teaching and learning in a new way.

In practical terms, it invites a constant questioning and revising of educational programs, curricula, health-care policies, institutional regulations (where one size fits all), assessment procedures, and use of only one form of "evidence." It leads us beyond nursing as a subset of medical sciences, while still being part of them and indeed merging and transcending them, but also informing them.

This leads to the question of what kind of curriculum can sustain such a *Caritas-Love Ethic* as an aspiration and inspiration?

> Our educational and epistemological and ethical
> models have to rise to the twenty-first-century occasion as a moral
> invitation and responsibility to create new or at least different
> educational and pedagogical options for science and society alike.
>
> (Watson, 2008a, p. 256)

A Caring Science/Caritas orientation to nursing education for now and our future intersects with arts and humanities and related fields of study, beyond the conventional, clinicalized and medicalized views of human and health-healing. For Nightingale, "[N]ursing involved a sense of presence higher than the human, a 'divine intelligence that creates, sustains, and organizes the universe—and our awareness of an inner connection with this higher reality'" (Macrae, 2001, quoted in Watson, 2005, p. 63). Her views, along with Levinas and his philosophy, invite us to "face our humanity" and our connectedness with the greater, infinite dimensions of our life and work.

In embarking upon a model of Caring Science/*Caritas* education, we invite others to create open space to allow an evolved/transformed human consciousness to enter our phenomenal field—opening to notions of *Caritas/Love and Infinity* of the human spirit and creativity beyond our imagination of today's standards (Levinas, 1969; Watson, 2005; Watson & Smith, 2002)

As we invite Love back into our hearts, our minds and our classrooms and our practices, we invite the originary Primordial Love back into all of life and all living things. For Levinas, and for us, this inviting Love back into our life, our work, our world, "is not meant to be anti-intellectual" (1969, p. 109) but rather to lead to the very development of intellect. Thus, this line of thinking makes a case for an underlying metaphysical-philosophical-ethical foundation for nursing rather than reverting to classical assumptions of science and knowledge and the technologies of teaching and learning. This view also reflects an evolutionary perspective for the nursing profession and the nature of knowledge itself.

> Nature and history are not just about the survival of the fittest,
> but also about the survival of the wisest . . . and the most aware.
>
> Ben Okri (1997, p. 133)

This evolution honors again the reality that having information is not necessarily knowledge, that knowledge by itself does not necessarily lead to understanding, and that understanding is not the same as wisdom or wisdom seeking (Watson, 2008b). As we reconsider nursing education within a broader ethos proposed here, we realize that our approaches to our learning and teaching and practices have been too small and limiting to allow for respect of the deeper aspects of our life and work. In other words, our jobs as educators have been too small with respect to the deep nature of the work of nurses and teachers, who are here to lift up the human spirit, to return to Love as foundation for being/becoming whole (Watson, 2008b). Thus, we extend a moral invitation to create new or at least different educational and pedagogical options for science and society alike.

> As we examine our truth of Belonging-Being-Knowing and Doing Caring-Healing work in the world, how can we any longer bear to sustain and perpetuate an empty, hollow model?
>
> Watson (2008b, p. 67)

AFFIRMATIONS OF CARING SCIENCE MINDSET FOR NURSING EDUCATION

- Every way of knowing becomes a way of living; thus, epistemology becomes ethic.
- Epistemology as ethic is a set of values to live by, a way to conduct our lives.
- Behind this reframed ethic is a way of knowing that is Personal.
- Truth is personal, radically personal, not abstract, at arm's length, propositional, "out there."
- Knowledge and knowing are communal; movement toward truth is a communal movement, with conflicts, dialogue, debates, and dialectical movement toward consensus.
- Truth emerges between and among us.
- Knowledge and knowing are about mutuality and reciprocity; truth seeks us from our heart-center, rather than us seeking truth

(Einstein talked about "listening to the universe speak"; there is a reciprocal dance between the knower and the knowing).

• Knowledge and knowing are transformational, in that knowledge and seeking knowing are being challenged toward truth seeking, toward changing one's life, causing one to live life more fully and deeply; waking to our connection with the larger universe.

• Knowing teaching, learning, and caring transform my knowing, teaching, and learning if they are guided by the images and norms of higher dimension consciousness.

The transformation-learning literature (Bache, 2001) has noted that words we use in teaching-learning, theories, and interpretations carry much power to influence others. Words not supported by the energy of personal experiences have much less power than words grounded in personal experiences that possess the energy of love and caring.

In this model, higher-energy thoughts such as Love and caring bring higher-frequency energy into the learning space, even if the space is nonlocal (Bache, 2001). Although the power of the teacher is critical to create the consciousness of a community of scholars and co-learners, the more important power is the power of the group, the community, the learning circle. Thus, the individual and collective involvement in one's own learning influences the strength and energetic stream that underpin the content (Bache, 2001; Watson, 2002).

The current intellectual revolutions in caring-healing-health knowledge and practices and Caring Science frameworks are right in front of us in society and science alike. We have to face the fact that whether we like it or not, whether we agree with it or not, there is evidence of an evolved global awareness of our shared humanity and our shared environment: the fact that we metaphorically and literally "hold another person's life in our hands." As nurse educators we are personally involved in transforming live encounters with the world through our scholarship, our knowledge, and our forms of teaching and learning—hence, a call for a new curriculum model, grounded, and informed/transformed through Caring Science as prevailing ethos and ethic.

Caring Science is not a unitary thing, a singular and rule-bound belief system. It engages with the diversity of the sciences and arts, philosophy, humanities, and with notions of personal growth, of transformative consciousness, learning by which the terms in which people think and the words they speak can actually be changed in educative situations. This takes time and trouble, or, put more forcefully, it takes a personal commitment by nurses to enliven the importance of human relationships and caring as the epicenter of what nursing actually means, as its first and necessary condition.

Such an approach applies also to our students so we can see their "faces" and our "faces" can be seen by them, and we are seen to practice what we teach. This is not easy. As noted, it takes a certain aspiration and inspiration, what is ultimately a metaphysical worldview that recognizes and accommodates the tensions that will be met along the way. This applies to both educator-student and student-educator, student-student relations. If we treat our relations with others merely as roles, there is a danger of collapsing back into a universally objectivist mode of thinking in which the educative relation has no face—this student, this lecturer, this patient, this nurse, this doctor, but no face, no "other," no unique individual. In the field of bioethics, these matters are often framed as issues of race, ethnicity, and power and so on (Watson, 2008b, p. 55).

From a Caring Science lens, Riane Eisler (2008b) makes a case for "caring economics," and the need for a "caring revolution" with respect to the values, politics, and policies of social-economic justice. She highlighted the fact that our economic values are guided toward reward, conquest, exploitation, and domination; this global political worldview toward social justice threatens the very survival of our species and our environment and spills over into our classrooms and our student-student, student-teacher, and teacher-to-teacher relationships.

Indeed the survival of humans and our planet is now up close and personal as never before with respect to these foundational issues that are embedded in the politics and economics of our globe.

> Thus, what is central in my role as a teacher to the student as other is responsibility. I have an obligation more primary than any freedom. In fact it might not be too strong to argue that my singularity as a teacher comes into existence through my exposure to the student as other. Here the otherness of the student can be characterized as uniqueness, something that transcends my categorization. The uniqueness of the student is actually a call to me for assuming responsibility to that person. I am responsible to her [sic] precisely because s/he is irreplaceable in the pedagogical relationship, regardless of how many others there are. At this moment, to that person,

I am responsible. That student, whose face I see, is irreplaceable, calling me to respond. This obligation is mine, personally.

(Joldersma, 2001, pp. 186–187)

Caring Science calls into question and offers a challenge to seek our way through the political, economic, and techno-rational infrastructures that increasingly weigh us down in the name of quality that searches for universal standards; whether in learning and teaching, research, administration, or curriculum planning and implementation. These same infrastructures also weigh on students in terms of assessments, progress reports, and research or project proposals.

There is no easy way out; we are all invited to enter into this new space together and cocreate what might be, rather than succumb to what is and no longer works for us, for students, for patients, for humanity. As we make this turn together, we can engage in some of the lingering questions that may serve as value and intellectual guides for curriculum reform/transformation.

Time Out for Reflection

How would you define a Caring Science curriculum?

What does Caring Science offer for nursing education and practice?

What is the difference between the discipline of nursing and the profession of nursing? Why is this difference important to understand?

What are the factors that distinguish a Caring Science curriculum from another type of nursing curriculum?

How can epistemology be/become an ethic?

How will you incorporate caring into your curriculum development process?

How can one justify having Love and Caring within its framework for education?

How would you describe issues of social-moral justice operating in your personal life world? Your experience as student, as student nurse?

PARTS AND WHOLES: THE RHETORICAL AND HAUNTING QUESTIONS FOR NURSING EDUCATION

There remains in nursing and science and society alike the rhetorical question about parts and wholes, Love and shared humanity, shared world. Although we are challenged to work with wholes, and whole human beings and whole knowledge systems, our dominant mythologies have tended to focus on parts. As such, there is an argument for wondering—are we to remain helpless and even destructive to ourselves and to our knowledge of human caring, healing, health, and humanity if we fail to ask and address the other side of the epistemological mythology?

We are ethically challenged to address new questions, especially for professional nursing education and curricula that invite wholes and Love and all of human experiences into our pedagogies and disciplinary knowledge matrix.

We each are invited to ponder the following rhetorical questions as a reflective self-guide toward transformative teaching and learning:

- How do we/you put the parts back into the whole?
- How do we/you integrate facts with meanings?
- How do we/you acknowledge that the personal is also the professional?
- How do we/you allow your/our ethics to become your/our epistemology rather than perpetuating epistemological myths that deform our ethics?
- How do we/you honor ontology-of-spirit-filled relationship and caring relationship as ethic, as epistemology, as pedagogy and praxis for advancing professional nursing and healing?
- How do we/you cocreate, develop, and practice Caring Science, rather than the dominant biomedical-technological science model?
- How do we create communities of caring in our classrooms and clinical settings?
- How do we create opportunities for authentic dialogue whereby all questions are considered sacred?
- How do we/you integrate, honor, and sustain humanity and relational *Human Caring-Love* in the midst of technological advances?

- How do we/you create a *Caritas curriculum and *Caritas Nurses for 21st century nursing and healing health care?

To take these questions another step, we offer some "Authentication Criteria for a Caring Science Curriculum"—

Philosophical and Operational Guidelines

In reviewing your current curriculum ask yourself, your system, and your curriculum the following questions:

> **Ethics:** Is there evidence in the curricular structure/organization/ content and teaching-learning experiences of an Universal Ethic of Caring? Is there evidence of experiences to learn Human Caring, starting with Self-Caring and radiating out in concentric circles to Other—Community—Environment—Planet—Universe?

Is there evidence of a cosmology of connectedness with All? Is it obvious that the worldview is such that it is understood that each person resides in a larger pattern of oneness with the environment/universe? This is framed as "Ethic of Belonging" to the universal field of infinite Cosmic Love (Levinas, see Watson, 2005).

- **Ontology:** Does the curriculum have evidence indicating that the development and implementation of the curriculum is based on the nature and substance of the discipline of nursing? That is: Are nursing philosophies, theories, research, and practice models of nursing phenomena and caring embedded within the curriculum throughout?

- **Epistemology:** Will the curriculum guide emancipatory pedagogies and teaching-learning patterns that engage students in all patterns and multiple ways of knowing within the discipline, congruent with, and located within, the domain of nursing and human phenomena?

- **Practice/Praxis:** Does the curriculum guide students to learn the practice of nursing from the perspective of nursing values, theories, and philosophies that incorporate caring and healing? Is there attention to helping the student to critique conventional practice? Is practice approached as Praxis? That is, practice that originates from

---

(***Authors' sidebar:** These questions were inspired and informed by Smith and McCarthy's criteria used to critique major nursing educational reports and recommendations for the future. [Smith & McCarthy, 2010] However, their criteria have been refined, extended, and transposed as philosophical and operational guides to creating a curriculum, grounded in an evolved disciplinary core of Caring Science.)

reflection, contemplation, and critique that is informed by the ethics, philosophies, values, and theories of caring and healing and human health illness phenomena?

- **Emancipatory Pedagogy:** Is there evidence of caring pedagogies as emancipatory learning experiences based upon faculty's consciousness of the need for meaningful personal and professional educational and practice experiences? Do faculty and curricular content, structure, relations, and learning experiences bring forth the missing dimension of health care, restoring the heart of nursing's disciplinary core of caring?

- **Teaching Learning Focus:** Does the curriculum guide the teaching-learning experience from the foundation of nursing's disciplinary knowledge, both intensively and extensively? (Smith & McCarthy, 2010, p. 46)? Is there evidence of honoring all the vicissitudes of the human condition for students/patients? Is there evidence of a passion for scholarship of the love of nursing? A love of humanity? Of self and other? A commitment for scholarship and knowledge of caring and healing embedded within the students' personal/professional relations and classroom/clinical experiences?

- **Differentiate Disciplinary Knowledge:** Does the curriculum orient the student to differentiate nursing's sphere of knowledge development from other disciplines and professions, especially medical science, through diverse forms of scholarly pursuit and critique?

- **Transdisciplinary Scholarship and Practices:** Is there evidence of respecting and incorporating other forms of knowledge and other professions within the sphere of learning and practice? Is it evident that Caring Science is transdisciplinary? Are there learning and teaching experiences and practices that demonstrate complementary, harmonious relations and learning with diverse theories, and fields of knowledge, science, and technology?

- **Social Justice and Equality:** Is there curricular evidence of classrooms and embodied experiences that demonstrate "communities of caring and equality"? Embracing and celebrating diversity, be it ideas, social, economic, gender, race, lifestyle, ethnicity, customs, and beliefs?

- **Caring Scholarship:** Is there evidence in the curriculum of scholarship that embraces multiple forms of inquiry toward research and creative work? Forms of Inquiry which contribute to generation of new disciplinary knowledge of nursing phenomena and human caring-healing-health?

We offer these reflective indicators of a Caring Science curriculum—an authentic intellectual blueprint and value-based guide for assessing present and future caring curricula that are grounded in the discipline of nursing. These guides represent "authentication criteria" and point toward new goals and standards for nursing as a mature and distinct human caring-healing-health discipline and profession.

As nursing education enters into this evolved disciplinary foundation to prepare the coming generations of nursing professionals, then it fully comes of age. Likewise, with this disciplinary foundation for nursing education, nursing will be sustaining its authentic commitment to, and Love of, humanity and the unknown, unfolding future. As it does so, it is positioned to fulfill its mission and covenant with society worldwide for the next 100 years.

We close with the words of Nigerian writer and poet Ben Okri and his perennial wisdom for our shared future:

> In a world like ours . . .
> . . . Individual authenticity lies in what we can find that is worth living for. And the only thing worth living for is Love . . . . The Love that can make us breathe again, Love a great and beautiful cause, a wonderful vision. A great Love for one another, or for the future.

Ben Okri (1997, p. 57)

REFERENCES

Bache, C. (2001). *Transformative learning*. Sausalito, CA: Noetic Sciences Institute.

Eisler, R. (2007) *The real wealth of nations: Creating a caring economics*. San Francisco: Berrett-Koehler.

Joldersma, C. W. (2001). *Pedagogy of the other: A levinasian approach to the student-teacher relationship. In philosophy of education yearbook*. Champaign, IL: University of Illinois at Urbana-Champaign.

Levinas, E. (1969). *Totality and infinity*. Pittsburgh, PA: Duquesne University. (14th printing, 2000).

Macrae, J. A. (2001). *Nursing as a spiritual practice*. New York: Springer.

Okri, B. (1997). *A way of being free*. London: Phoenix.

Palmer, P. (2004). *The violence of our knowledge: Toward a spirituality of higher education. 21st learning initiative*. Kalamazoo, MI: Fetzer Institute.

Smith, M., & McCarthy, P. (2010) Disciplinary knowledge in nursing education: Going beyond the blueprint. *Nursing Outlook, 58*(10), 44–51.

Watson, J. (2002). Metaphysics of virtual caring communities. *International Journal of Human Caring, 6*(1), 41–45.

Watson, J. (2005). *Caring science as sacred science.* Philadelphia: FA Davis.

Watson, J. (2008a). *Nursing. The philosophy and science of caring.* New Revised Edition. Boulder, CO: University Press of Co.

Watson, J. (2008b). Social justice and human caring: A model of caring science as a hopeful paradigm for moral justice for humanity. *Creative Nursing Journal, 14*(2), 54–61.

Watson, J., & Smith, M. (2002). Caring science and the science of unitary human beings: A transtheoretical discourse. *Journal of Advanced Nursing, 37*(5), 452–461.

INDEX